The Handbook of Forensic Rehabilitation

William H. Burke, Ph.D., Editor

HDI Publishers
P.O. Box 131401
Houston, Texas, 77219

Design and layout by Sharon Roeske and J. Charles Haynes.

Printed in the United States of America.

This book is printed on acid-free paper. ∞

Library of Congress Cataloging-in-Publication Data
The handbook of forensic rehabilitation / William H. Burke, editor.
p. cm.
Includes bibliographical references and index.
ISBN 1-882855-31-0
1. Medical rehabilitation--Handbooks, manuals, etc. 2. Medical rehabilitation--Law and legislation--United States--Handbooks, manuals, etc. I. Burke, William H., 1948-
RM930.H348 1994
614'.1--dc20 94-41909
CIP

To Rebecca and Katie,
my support and inspiration

THE HANDBOOK OF FORENSIC REHABILITATION

Contents

List of Tables

List of Figures

About the Editor

William H. Burke, Ph.D., CRC

William H. Burke, Ph.D., CRC is the Clinical Director of Optimal Environments, a community-based neurologic rehabilitation and supported independent living program in Tampa, Florida. Dr. Burke also maintains a Forensic Rehabilitation practice with offices in New Hampshire and Florida. Recognized internationally for his expertise in the field of Brain Injury rehabilitation, Dr. Burke designed and developed three of the earliest residential, post hospital Brain Injury rehabilitation centers in the U.S. and today he consults with Brain Injury rehabilitation centers throughout the country. Over the past 10 years Dr. Burke has treated over 1200 Brain and Spinal Injury patients. His earlier professional activities include 15 years in the field of rehabilitation as a clinician, administrator and university professor. Dr. Burke consults throughout the U.S. and Canada with attorneys, insurance companies and government agencies to develop comprehensive rehabilitation and life long plans of care in Brain and Spinal Injury cases.

Dr. Burke is a well known author in the field of Brain Injury rehabilitation and lectures on the topic nationally. He is the senior editor of *Rehabilitation and Treatment of Traumatic Brain Injury*, a 20-volume set of books regarding Brain Injury rehabilitation. He has authored and published over 40 research articles and outcome studies on Brain Injury and contributed chapters to two recent text books, *Innovations in Head Injury Rehabilitation* and *Cognitive Rehabilitation in Perspective*. Dr. Burke is a member of the editorial review board for the *Journal of Rehabilitation*, and is on the Editorial Advisory Board of *The Neurolaw Letter*. He is an active member of the National Head Injury Foundation, serving on its Education and Training Committee and Task Force on Life Long Care.

Dr. Burke received his Ph.D. in Rehabilitation from the Florida State University and a M.A. in Rehabilitation Counseling from the University of South Florida. He is a Certified Rehabilitation Counselor (CRC), licensed in the Commonwealth of Massachusetts and is a Diplomate of The American Board of Professional Disability Consultants.

Contributors

Kenneth N. Anchor, Ph.D., ABPP
Associate Professor of Psychology and Human Development, Vanderbilt University.

Bruce L. Bird, Ph.D.
Licensed Psychologist and Executive Director of the Institutes for Behavior Resources, Washington, DC.

Heidi Fawber, M.Ed., CRC
Rehabilitation Case Manager and Program Coordinator, Outpatient Head Injury Services, Harmerville Rehabilitation Center, Pittsburgh, PA.

Sheldon Margulies, M.D., J.D.
Assistant Professor, Department of Neurology, University of Maryland and Johns Hopkins University. Dr. Margulies maintains a private practice in Silver Spring, MD.

Barbara Z. Orstein., M.Ed., CRC
Rehabilitation Case Manager in Private Practice, Harrisburgh, PA.

David R. Price, Ph.D.
Founder and President of the Insurance/Defense Network, Greenville, SC.

Debra C. Price, Ph.D.
Licensed Counseling Psychologist and Senior Case Analyst with the Insurance/Defense Network, Greenville, SC.

David E. Raskin, M.D.
Clinical Professor of Psychiatry, Jefferson Medical College of Philadelphia. Dr. Raskin maintains his private practice in Wilmington, DE.

Carole W. Sellars, Ph.D.
Founder and Coordinator of the Pediatric Brain Injury Program at Gillette Children's Hospital, St. Paul, MN.

Linda R. Shaw, Ph.D., CRC
Assistant Professor of Rehabilitation Counseling, University of Florida, and current President of the American Rehabilitation Counseling Association.

Harold H. Smith, Ph.D., ABPP
Neuropsychologist in Private Practice, Largo, FL.

Jerome M. Staller, Ph.D.
Founder and Director of Center for Forensic Economic Studies, Philadelphia, PA

Lawrence R. Tancredi, M.D., J.D.
Psychiatrist in private practice in New York City.

THE HANDBOOK OF FORENSIC REHABILITATION

Foreword

Forensic Rehabilitation has evolved over the last three decades. The roots of this specialization can be traced back to legislation that mandated medical and vocational rehabilitation of injured workers. This mandate gave rise to the privatization of rehabilitation. Private rehabilitation was initially organized by rehabilitation and medical practitioners with the goal of returning Worker's Comp claimants to their former jobs. While this aspect of forensic rehabilitation has grown significantly over the past twenty-five years, this specialization has further evolved during the last ten years into the courtroom. Currently, medical and rehabilitation practitioners are routinely involved as experts in third-party litigation. Rehabilitation and medical experts were introduced into the litigation arena primarily by plaintiff counsel in an effort to justify damages. However, defense counsel and insurance claims executives quickly responded and have begun to routinely seek the assistance of forensic experts as well.

Forensic Rehabilitation quite simply is the application of rehabilitation, medical and economic principles to the legal system and insurance industry. In the legal arena, forensic rehabilitation experts work together to analyze the extent to which a person has been injured or disabled, to determine the etiology of the individual's disabilities, to estimate damages and to provide expert testimony. In the insurance arena, forensic rehabilitation experts often provide claims management and case management in addition to the above legal oriented activities. This text is designed to serve as a "handbook" for medical and rehabilitation professionals, claims professionals, as well as plaintiff and defense counsel. The concepts and strategies presented in this volume can be applied to a wide variety of cases; however, this text purposely emphasizes the claims of brain injury and psychological injury due to the volume and monetary implications of these cases.

This text is organized into twelve chapters that have been authored by nationally recognized experts in the field of forensic and medical rehabilitation. The first chapter provides an overview and history of forensic rehabilitation. In this chapter, Dr. Shaw traces the roots of forensic rehabilitation over the past seventy-five years of development through legislation that initially established rehabilitation services in the United States and gave rise to private sector rehabilitation. Ultimately she discusses the introduction of medical and rehabilitation activities in third-party litigation. Dr. Shaw also offers insights regarding the future of forensic rehabilitation. She notes that the current insurance-driven system is expected to undergo a number of changes over the coming years, particularly in light of the current emphasis on health care reform.

Central to the field of forensic rehabilitation is the role of the rehabilitation expert. Chapter two presents an overview of the role and function of the rehabilitation expert in the analysis and management of brain injury and other neurologic disorders. In this chapter, Dr. Burke presents a unique and contemporary model of rehabilitation management: rehabilitation triage. The goals of this process are to improve each individual's level of function while reducing their need for assistance through the development of specialized rehabilitation and life care plans. Case examples are provided in this chapter that demonstrate the utility of this rehabilitation triage model as a method of managing claims and estimating damages in neurologic injury cases.

Another critical aspect of forensic rehabilitation is the analysis of the injured individual's claim. In chapter three, Dr. Price presents a comprehensive method of case analysis which utilizes the multi-axial differential diagnosis methodology recently revised in the DSM-IV. This method of analysis includes a comprehensive evaluation of an individual's pre-existing level of function as well as presenting methods to differentiate organic versus psychiatric etiology to explain an individual's current status. This chapter provides an excellent yet brief overview that will assist attorneys and claims professionals to better understand the newly revised DSM-IV diagnostic system.

Lost access to the labor market and lost future earning capacity are extremely important when estimating damages and/or setting reserves following an injury. Chapter four outlines the role of the vocational consultant in forensic rehabilitation. This chapter presents an overview of vocational evaluation and discusses methods of projecting future earning potential. Dr. Anchor also presents a brief description of vocational economics.

Case Management has developed over the past twenty years as an integral part of the rehabilitation of disabled individuals. In chapter five, Ms. Fawber and Ms. Orstein discuss the emergence of specialty case management in forensic rehabilitation. Forensic case management provides assistance to both plaintiff and defense counsel as the case is prepared for litigation. The role and function of forensic case managers as facilitators, coordinators, educators, problem-solvers and cost containment specialists are discussed. This chapter also outlines the benefits of specialized case management as a method of claims management.

Claims of mild head injury and/or post-concussion syndrome are increasingly encountered by both claims professionals, plaintiff counsel and defense counsel. In chapter six, Dr. Bird presents methods to analyze and manage claims of mild head injury in forensic rehabilitation. Dr. Bird provides an extensive review of the current literature regarding diagnosis, treatment and outcome of mild head injury. This chapter also provides the reader with methods to accurately diagnose or dispute claims of mild head injury. In addition, this chapter provides treatment guidelines when in fact diagnosis of mild head injury or post-concussion syndrome has been confirmed.

Children with brain injuries present the forensic rehabilitation specialist with a unique challenge. Chapter seven presents an overview of current epidemiological data, outcome research and financial information regarding pediatric brain injury. In this chapter, Drs. Sellars and Burke present methods of developing rehabilitation and life care plans specific to infants and children with acquired brain injury.

Medical examination by qualified neurologists and psychiatrists provide important information to assist forensic rehabilitation specialists in analyzing a patient's current status and future needs. In chapter eight, Dr. Margulies describes the mechanisms of brain injury, provides an overview of neuroimaging techniques, and discusses the importance of the face-to-face neurologic examination.

In addition to neurologic examination, psychiatric examination provides the forensic rehabilitation specialist with the data necessary to distinguish organic versus functional etiology in relation to an individual's complaints. In chapter nine, Drs. Raskin and Tancredi discuss the importance of the forensic psychiatric examination versus the clinical psychiatric examination to distinguish psychiatric disorders that are related to an injury or trauma from disorders that pre-existed the injury or have developed over time.

While neurologic and psychiatric examination are extremely important in forensic rehabilitation, the neuropsychological examination is uniquely sensitive to identifying particularly subtle brain injury. Dr. Smith, in chapter ten, discusses the specifics of the neuropsychological examination and offers suggestions to attorneys and claims professionals in selecting a neuropsychologist. In addition, this chapter presents an overview of the neuropsychological tests that will assist the non-neuropsychologist in interpreting neuropsychological reports.

In many cases of personal injury, industrial injury, product liability and medical malpractice, the question of malingering and/or secondary gain is bound to arise. In chapter eleven, Drs. Price, Raskin and Price present an overview of malingering and specifically discuss methods for the identification of and/or to rule out malingering as an explanation of an individual's disabilities. Methods of differential diagnosis to confirm or eliminate malingering as an explanation of an individual's current presentation are reviewed.

Finally, the "bottom line" in this emerging field of forensic rehabilitation is placing the monetary value on an injury. Dr. Staller discusses economic analysis in forensic rehabilitation emphasizing the importance of the economist as a member of the forensic rehabilitation team. In chapter twelve, Dr. Staller discusses the elements of damages including medical costs, lost earning capacity, and presents methods of economic analysis to determine the total economic loss over the lifetime of an injured person.

The publication of this text was made possible by the diligent efforts of many people. To each author I want to express my sincere appreciation for the time, energy and insight they devoted to this project. I also want to express my appreciation for the direct and indirect assistance of my colleagues, mentors, and teachers who helped to shape my values and perspectives over the years. Finally, I want to say thank you to my assistant, Carol Jaques. Without her dedicated assistance, this text would not have become a reality.

WHB, 1995

THE HANDBOOK OF FORENSIC REHABILITATION

1

FORENSIC REHABILITATION: HISTORICAL AND FUTURE PERSPECTIVES

Linda R. Shaw, Ph.D., CRC

This chapter will trace the social and legal roots of the field of forensic rehabilitation and speculate on the future of forensic rehabilitation in light of current legal economic and social issues.

State-Federal Vocational Rehabilitation

The need for an "expert" in the vocational rehabilitation of persons with disabilities was created by a series of legislative acts which established a vocational rehabilitation program for persons with disabilities.

TABLE 1. 1 *Rehabilitation Legislation*

1918	SMITH-SEARS ACT (SOLDIERS' REHABILITATION ACT) P.L. 178	Established vocational retraining program for disabled veterans
1920	SMITH-FESS ACT (CIVILIAN VOCATIONAL ACT) P.L. 236	First Civilian rehabilitation program; emphasis on vocational retraining
1936	RANDOLPH-SHEPPARD ACT	Established vending stands operated by persons who are blind
1943	BARDON-LaFOLLETTE ACT P.L. 78-113	Provision of medical, surgical, and other restorative services

TABLE 1.1 *Rehabilitation Legislation, continued*

1954	VOCATIONAL REHABILITATION ACT AMENDMENTS P.L. 83-565	Federal support of training personnel in rehabilitation; of research & demonstration projects; established funding for vocational evaluation
1965	VOCATIONAL REHABILITATION ACT AMENDMENTS P.L. 89-333	Increased services to persons with severe disabilities, mental retardation, sensory impairments, and behavior disorders; financial aid for training of personnel extended
1965	SOCIAL SECURITY ACT AMENDMENTS P.L. 89-97	Extended vocational rehabilitation services to Social Security Disability Insurance recipients
1973	VOCATIONAL REHABILITATION ACT AMENDMENTS P.L. 93-113	Major civil rights legislation discrimination in federal hiring, addressed accessibility standards, affirmative action, and equal opportunity; established priority on serving severely disabled and client involvement and advocacy
1975	EDUCATION OF ALL HANDICAPPED CHILDREN ACT P.L. 94-142	Intended to ensure mainstreaming and quality special education
1978	VOCATIONAL REHABILITATION ACT AMENDMENTS P.L. 95-602	Funded grants for Independent Living Programs; established the National Institute of Handicapped Research and the National Council on Handicapped
1990	THE AMERICANS WITH DISABILITIES ACT P.L. 101-336	Prohibited discrimination against qualified individuals in employment; prohibits discrimination by public accommodations; mandates telecommunications relay services

Table 1.1 summarizes several of the acts which established and impacted the ongoing development of the program, starting with the 1918 Soldiers Rehabilitation Act and concluding with the 1992 Rehabilitation Act Amendments. This legislation established a precedent for the provision of vocational rehabilitation services which was later adopted by many states' workers' compensation programs. The new agency created by the early legislation was staffed with persons from a variety of professional fields, many of them from education. However, as the complexity of the services offered increased and the scope of persons served expanded, it became apparent that a new professional discipline was required—one which would consist of professionals trained in disability, counseling, case management, vocational evaluation, and placement. Consequently, the 1954 amendments to the Vocational Rehabilitation Act (P.L. 83-565) provided funding to establish graduate programs in rehabilitation counseling. The profession developed gradually; however, the demand for masters prepared rehabilitation counselors continued to outstrip supply, resulting in the state programs hiring "counselors" who did not possess masters degrees. Indeed, in some states, the only qualification was a high school diploma. Deutsch (1983) notes that it was not until the early 1970s that a certification program guided by the Commission on Rehabilitation Counselor Certification was established to assure a minimum standard of competency.

Social Security Disability Insurance Program

The State-Federal Vocational Rehabilitation Program established an important backdrop for the development of the role of the vocational expert in that it created a demand for professionals who possessed the unique skills and training which would eventually become necessary for the vocational expert. In many respects, however, the advent of forensic rehabilitation can be directly traced to the establishment of the Social Security Disability Insurance (SSDI) Program. This program was legislated into existence in 1954 and a few years later was modified to allow the disbursement of actual cash benefits for persons whose disability was deemed severe enough to prevent them from working (Harper, 1985). Not surprisingly, disputes soon arose when claimants, who believed their injuries precluded gainful employment, were denied benefits. An appeals system was established for persons whose claims had been denied. In such cases, the Social Security Administration (SSA) was confronted with the dilemma of producing evidence to justify its assertion that the payment of disability benefits was not justified.

The SSA's burden of proof became "heavier" in 1960 when a decision by the U.S. Court of Appeals held that in those cases where it had been clearly established that an individual could not return to his/her former occupation, the SSA must determine the other kinds of work in which the individual could engage. This decision prompted the SSA in 1962 to establish criteria for employing vocational experts to provide testimony on the availability of jobs for which the claimant was suitable. The criteria included the following:

A. Recent Experience
   1. Rehabilitation counseling and/or placement, particularly with clients having prior work experience.
   2. The use of occupational materials developed for vocational counseling, including information about the requirements such as duties, skills, physical demands, working conditions, and occupationally significant characteristics. A working knowledge of the <u>Dictionary of Occupational Titles</u> and its supplements are important.
   3. The utilization of the concept of transferability of skills in terms of worker traits and functions.

B. Ability to observe and evaluate personal characteristics, educational, and vocational background.

C. Well rounded, up-to-date knowledge of, and experience with, industrial and occupational trends and local labor market conditions (Harper, 1985, p. 56-57).

The only professional discipline which encompassed this particular set of skills and knowledge was rehabilitation counseling, the product of the State-Federal Vocational Rehabilitation system. Increasingly, vocational rehabilitation counselors were called upon to provide their expert opinions regarding claimants' employability.

As Harper (1985) notes, many claimants were represented by attorneys who gained ample first hand evidence of the benefits of the information a vocational expert could bring to a case. In the increasing number of cases where the claimants had attorney representation, the vocational experts found themselves subject to close cross-examination. Consequently, they began to develop and hone their skills, carefully documenting their testimony. This early exposure of the vocational expert and attorneys to one another foreshadowed the attorney's use of the vocational expert as an expert witness in other venues and areas of legal practice. As Harper (1985) notes , "It was only natural that the attorneys and the vocational evaluators would eventually form an alliance which would result in a more effective presentation of loss of earning capacity in personal-injury litigation (p. 57). The use of the vocational expert in social security cases diminished considerably with the introduction of the medical-vocational grid which provided for disability rulings based upon objective factors such as age, education and medical factors characterizing the claimant (Field, Weed & Grimes, 1986). As Rasch (1985) notes, the role of the vocational expert in Social Security cases is considerably more limited than that with Workers' Compensation or personal injury cases. Within the Social Security system, vocational experts must follow set guidelines in developing opinions (p. 158). As Grenfell (1980) noted, the use of vocational experts by the SSA rose steadily in the 1960s and 1970s. However, in 1980, the SSA drastically reduced the number of vocational experts under contract as a cost-saving measure. While the role of vocational experts within the Social Security system is somewhat diminished today, the early involvement of vocational rehabilitation counselors and evaluators within this system established an important precedent. The recognition by attorneys of the value of expert vocational testimony set the stage for the rapid development of the role of the vocational expert.

Private Sector Rehabilitation

Most observers of the advent of forensic rehabilitation agree that the specialty, as we define it today, could not have developed without the privatization movement within the field of rehabilitation counseling. The privatization of rehabilitation occurred in response to the ongoing development of the Workers' Compensation system in America, most especially, the inclusion of mandatory vocational rehabilitation services as a covered benefit. Concurrently with the development of services to people with disabilities in other sectors, the Workers' Compensation system developed slowly over the first half of the century on a state-by-state basis. As Matkin (1986) notes, "The principle underlying Workers' Compensation is that industrialization benefits everyone in society and since injury and death are inevitable in industrial activity, everyone in society should help bear the economic consequences" (p. 37). According to the U.S. Chamber of Commerce, the objectives of Workers' Compensation are as follows:

A. "provide sure, prompt and reasonable income and medical benefits for work-related accidents, or income benefits to their dependents, regardless of fault;
B. provide a single remedy and reduce court delays, costs and work loads arising out of personal injury litigation;
C. relieve public and private charities of financial drains;
D. eliminate payment of fees to lawyers and witnesses as well as time-consuming trials and appeals;
E. encourage maximum employer interest in safety and rehabilitation through appropriate experience rating mechanism, and;
F. promote frank study of causes of accidents rather than concealment of fault." (p. vii)
(U.S. Chamber of Commerce, 1984)

While these objectives were intended to apply to all of the states' programs, there existed wide variation from state to state in the degree to which the states were effective in meeting these goals, particularly, the need to address safety issues in the workplace (Bowers & Bursinger, 1986). Consequently, in 1970 the U.S. Congress passed the Occupational Safety and Health Act (OSHA). One section of OSHA established the National Commission for State Workers' Compensation Laws, charged with determining the effectiveness of each state's Workers' Compensation system. The work of this Commission resulted in 119 recommendations. While vocational rehabilitation issues were not prominent among these recommendations, the work of the Commission resulted in an awareness among the states of their differences, one of which was the extent to which rehabilitation services were mandated. Since 1916, New York State had provided for vocational rehabilitation of the injured workman. Several states had mandatory rehabilitation and many others contained provisions for vocational rehabilitation. Still others had no provisions for rehabilitation within the Workers' Compensation system, and instead relied upon the state-federal vocational rehabilitation system to supply injured workers with rehabilitation services. As a result of the increased awareness brought about by the Commission's work, coupled with an increasing dissatisfaction with the state-federal system's ability to quickly return claimants to work, the states began enacting provisions to include rehabilitation services in one form or another. By 1976, 27 states had some type of vocational rehabilitation; and during the late 1970s and early 1980s, many additional states enacted mandatory vocational rehabilitation laws. Others began to allow for expenses associated with vocational rehabilitation in their policies determining the amounts of lump sum settlements (Gann & Moreland, 1992).

The role of the rehabilitation counselor within such systems generally involves vocational evaluation to establish eligibility, case management, and placement services. As with the SSDI program, however, attorneys representing claimants who had been denied their Workers' Compensation claims began to call upon vocational specialists to provide expert opinions regarding employability.

Again, the rehabilitation counselor found him/herself cast in this new role—that of expert witness.

Insurance Rehabilitation

The rise of private sector rehabilitation is directly related to the costs associated with the Workers' Compensation system. Weed and Field (1990) note that, "With rising costs of medical expenses and payment of lost wages for industrially injured, a number of companies began to look at possible ways to contain costs as well as to have more control over vocational rehabilitation of injured workers. Many insurance companies found that state rehabilitation counselors were placing injured workers into two or more years of training, thereby obligating insurance carriers to continue compensation payments until clients had completed training programs" (p. 4). Insurance companies began to hire and to contract with rehabilitation "specialists" to contain costs. Such personnel included rehabilitation nurses to oversee medical management, and rehabilitation counselors to effect a speedy and cost-effective return to work (Matkin, 1982; Shrey, 1979). The 70's witnessed a revolution in the field of rehabilitation counseling. The for-profit rehabilitation industry boomed from being literally nonexistent in 1970 to an industry comprised of nearly 1,000 companies in 1982 with revenues near $25 million (Lauterbach, 1982).

The role of the rehabilitation counselors in insurance rehabilitation was very similar to that of rehabilitation counselors employed elsewhere, including vocational assessment, medical management, job development, and placement (Matkin, 1983; McMahon & Matkin, 1983). As Brandon (1983) noted, however, "one exception to traditional services looms impressively in this emerging model, and that is the role of litigation for the rehabilitationist. For those individuals in both the public and private sectors, litigation comes with the territory when working with the industrially injured workers. . . . It comes as no surprise, then, that the vocational rehabilitation specialist who has been working the entire spectrum of services with the industrially injured worker is now being discovered and employed as an expert witness in third party litigation" (p. 103).

Third-Party Litigation

The advent of third party litigation (primarily personal injury, products liability, and medical malpractice litigation) has had a significant impact on the field of rehabilitation (Deutsch, 1990). Emener (1986) referred to the 1980s as the "Era of Litigation" and noted that "the field of rehabilitation most assuredly has been influenced by this social zeitgeist" (p. 60).

May (1983) considered the increased use of vocational expert testimony in third party cases to be inevitable. He observed that:

> Because of the impact these [vocational expert] witnesses had on these early Social Security disability hearings, the concept of the vocational expert witness soon spread to other legal settings that included industrial hearings (workers compensation, personal injury, product liability, and divorce). . . . However, due to [the] increase in the number of private practitioners, the market for vocational experts in industrial and Social Security hearings has become highly competitive and somewhat overcrowded. It is not surprising then that the vocational rehabilitation expert witness should turn to other markets for vocational services, and not rely so heavily on markets where increasing competition has made them less lucrative." (p. 100)

In point of fact, personal injury and product liability expert witness work is far more profitable, and considered by many as a wide open, very lucrative field of practice for rehabilitation counselors.

The focus of the vocational expert's testimony in personal injury cases has historically been the impact of the injury on the individual's future earning capacity. Harper (1985) observes that "you are being asked to estimate in dollars and cents what an individual can earn or be trained to earn after their injury or if they are employable at all" (p. 59). Deutsch (1985) notes that the courts have gradually evolved in their awareness that there is no simple way to predict damages resulting from an injury based solely on medical testimony. Deutsch maintains that "static" awards based on current earnings were increasingly seen as unfair and unrealistic, given rapidly changing economic conditions. He asserts that "jurors want an 'authority' for statements that an individual's income will increase over time, that the average worker can be expected to work a given number of years, that an individual with specific physiological problems is indeed precluded from doing the same job that he had been doing before his accident, etc." (p. 100). Additionally, there has been an increasing awareness of the need to establish damages not only in terms of lost income potential but in terms of the additional <u>costs</u> the injured party will incur as a direct result of the injury. Consequently, in addition to determining lost earning capacity, the rehabilitation expert has increasingly been called upon to render an opinion about the predicted lifetime costs of such things as the cost of replacing household services the injured person can no longer perform, personal care, projected medical expenses, medical equipment and supplies, rehabilitation services, and vocational retraining (Deutsch, 1983). In order to assist rehabilitation experts in preparing for this expanded and complex role, Deutsch and Sawyer (1990) published a landmark text entitled "A Guide to Rehabilitation". This text ushered in the advent of "Life Care Planning," a systematic process of estimating damages based upon factual verifiable economic data coupled with the vocational experts' evaluative skills and rehabilitation knowledge.

Initially, rehabilitation experts in personal injury litigation cases were primarily utilized by the plaintiff's attorney. However, defense attorneys soon discovered that they could utilize rehabilitation experts to evaluate the fairness of the damages estimated by the plaintiff's expert witness. Today, rehabilitation experts are being utilized in personal injury cases in increasing numbers. Books and seminars abound educating attorneys about the advantages of retaining rehabilitation experts and rehabilitation professionals on the fine points of developing life care plans and providing testimony. (Deutsch, Sawyer, Jenkins, & Kitchen, 1986; Deutsch, Weed,

Kitchen, & Sluis, 1989; Weed & Riddick, 1992).

Future Focus

Forensic rehabilitation cannot help but be influenced by the social and legal influences impacting health care and the legal system today. The continued high cost of health care will undoubtedly result in systemic changes, the exact nature of which are difficult to predict. What is certain, however, is that the current insurance-driven system will undergo changes within the next several years. Health care reform is an ongoing process and the system is likely to remain in a state of evolution for many years, although change is likely to occur at an unprecedented pace. Those with a stake in expert testimony would do well to attend carefully to the changes which are sure to affect their role and the opportunities available to them.

The recent sentiment among some which favors legislation capping punitive awards in personal injury and malpractice litigation may eventually affect the degree to which attorneys will consider the hiring of rehabilitation experts to be desirable. Again, rehabilitation experts will need to carefully monitor such trends.

Professionalization

As the specialty of the rehabilitation expert continues to develop, a concern with professional identity has arisen. As the role of the Rehabilitation Expert has become increasingly specialized, many professionals engaged in forensic work have voiced concerns that the traditional university training programs and professional associations in rehabilitation counseling no longer seem attuned to their needs. Gamboa, Holland, and Tierney (1988) note that in the absence of support for the creation of divisions for rehabilitation and vocational experts within such professional associations as the American Counseling Association (ACA) and the National Rehabilitation Association (NRA), many experts have gravitated toward several new professional associations that have formed.

These include the National Association of Forensic Economists (NAFE), which is comprised of both vocational experts and economists; and the American Vocational Economic Association (AVEA), a nonprofit association, whose membership also includes both vocational experts and economists.

Opportunities

At this pivotal point in the history of health care, it is difficult to make any predictions about the directions in which this specialty will move with any degree of certainty. However, one can speculate about several areas in which rehabilitation experts have already become involved and in which the opportunities seem likely to expand. These include:

A. *Divorce* - Vocational experts are currently utilized to develop vocational plans and to determine the costs of necessary training for use in determining divorce settlements. This trend is expected to continue (May, 1983).
B. *Victims of Abuse* - Vocational experts are increasingly being utilized in determining damages for reduced employability and psychological treatment for battered women and victims of abuse (Choppa & Shafer, 1992).
C. *Discrimination Suits* - Vocational experts are increasingly finding a market for their skills in several kinds of discrimination cases. Passage of the Civil Rights Amendments of 1991 will likely result in an increase in discrimination cases filed in the civil court. With the passage of the ADA, vocational experts will particularly find a market for their expertise in determining a plaintiff's qualifications to perform the job in question, evaluating the employer's attempts to make reasonable accommodation and other related issues (McMahon & Shaw, 1992). The AIDS epidemic virtually insures that persons diagnosed with AIDS and HIV will be increasingly well-represented among plaintiffs alleging discrimination. Additionally, as

the baby boom generation matures, there will likely be an increase in age discrimination cases. Such cases are well within the purview of the vocational expert. The effect of sexual harassment on earning capacity will also likely receive increased attention in the courts (Choppa & Shafer, 1992) and vocational experts may play a key role in assessing damages.

SUMMARY

The role of the rehabilitation expert has steadily evolved over the past several decades with its roots in the state-federal rehabilitation system. The specialty began to "come into its own" with the emergence of the Social Security Disability Insurance program. The role of the rehabilitation expert has developed and changed in response to the various venues in which the expert's testimony has been utilized, including the workers' compensation system and third party litigation.

The future of forensic rehabilitation appears healthy with new opportunities and expanded roles being created by the social and legal trends of the 90's. Rehabilitation experts are finding a role in divorce, discrimination, and other civil cases. While those involved in or interested in pursuing rehabilitation expert work should feel optimistic about the field, they should carefully monitor the imminent changes likely in the health care field. A trend toward increased specialization and a distinct professional identity appears to be emerging and is likely to gain momentum as the opportunities for the rehabilitation expert expands.

REFERENCES

Boviers, C. & Bursinger, K.L. (1986). A history and overview of the Workers' Compensation System. *Journal of Private Sector Rehabilitation,* 1(2), 83-86.

Brandon, T.L. (1983). Vocational rehabilitation specialists in the courtroom. *Vocational Evaluation and Work Adjustment Bulletin,* 16(3), 103-108.

Choppa, A.J. & Shafer, K. (1992). Introduction to personal injury and expert witness work. In J.M. Siefker (Ed.). *Vocational Evaluation in Private Sector Rehabilitation,* 130-168. Menomonie, WI: Materials Development Center, Stout Vocational Rehabilitation Institute.

Deutsch, P.M. (1990). *A Guide to Rehabilitation Testimony: The Expert's Role as an Educator.* Orlando, FL: PMD Press, Inc.

Deutsch, P.M. & Raffa, F.A. (1983). *Damages in Tort Actions, Volume 8.* New York, NY: Matthew Bender.

Deutsch, P.M. & Sawyer, H.W. (1990). *A Guide to Rehabilitation.* New York, NY: Matthew Bender.

Deutsch, P., Sawyer, H., Jenkins, W. & Kitchen, J. (1986). Life care planning in catastrophic case management. *Journal of Private Sector Rehabilitation,* 1(1), 13-27.

Deutsch, P., Weed, R., Kitchen, J. & Sluis, A. (1989). *Life Care Plans for the Head Injured: A Step by Step Guide.* Orlando, FL: PMD Press.

Emener, W.G. (1986). Future perspectives on rehabilitation in America. *Journal of Private Sector Rehabilitation..* 1(2), 59-70.

Field, T.F., Weed. R.O., and Grimes, J.W. (1986). *The Vocational Expert Handbook.* Tuscon, AZ: Valpar International Corp.

Gamboa, A.M., Holland, G.H. & Tierney, J.P. (1988). Assessing work and earning capacity. *Advances in Clinical Rehabilitation,* 2, 6-36.

Gann, C. & Moreland, T. (1992). Introduction to insurance and workers' compensation. In J.M. Siefker (Ed.). *Vocational evaluation in private sector rehabilitation*, 67-98. Menomonie, WI: Materials Development Center, Stout Vocational Rehabilitation Institute.

Grenfell, J.G. (1980). The attorney use of a vocational expert. In *How to profitably handle Social Security cases.* Indianapolis, IN: Indiana Continuing Legal Education Forum.

Harper, R.B. (1985). The rehabilitation counselor as an expert witness in personal-injury litigation. In L.J. Taylor, M. Golter, G. Golter, & T.E. Backer (Eds.). *Handbook of Private Sector Rehabilitation,* 55-69. New York, NY: Springer Publishing Co.

Lauterback, J.R. (1982). Coaching the disabled back to work. *Industry Week,* April 5, 52-55.

Matkin, R. (1982). Rehabilitation services offered in the private sector: A pilot investigation. *Journal of Rehabilitation,* 48(4), 31-33.

Matkin, R.E. (1983). The roles and functions of rehabilitation specialists in the private sector. *Journal of Applied Rehabilitation Counseling,* 14(1), 14-27.

Matkin, R.E. (1986). *Insurance Rehabilitation.* Austin, TX: Pro-Ed.

May, V.R., III (1983). The vocational expert witness: Expanding the market place. *Vocational Evaluation and Work Adjustment Bulletin,* 16(3), 100-102.

McMahon, B. & Matkin, R. (1983). Pre-service graduate education for private sector rehabilitation counselors. *Rehabilitation Counseling Bulletin,* 27, 54-60.

Rasch, J. (1985). *Rehabilitation of Workers' Compensation and Other Insurance Claimants.* Springfield, IL: Charles C. Thomas.

Shrey, D. (1979). The rehabilitation counselor in industry: A new frontier. *Journal of Applied Rehabilitation Counseling,* 9(4), 168-172.

United States Chamber of Commerce (1984). *Analysis of Workers Compensation Laws.* Washington, DC: Author.

Weed, R.O. & Field, T.F. (1990). *Rehabilitation Consultant's Handbook.* Athens, GA: Elliott & Fitzpatrick, Inc.

Weed, R.O. & Reddick, S.N. (1992). Life care plans as a case management tool. *The Case Manager*, 3(1), 26-35.

Linda R. Shaw, Ph.D., CRC

Dr. Shaw is an Assistant Professor in the Department of Rehabilitation Counseling at the University of Florida. She is currently the President of the American Rehabilitation Counseling Association and is active in several professional associations. Dr. Shaw has published and presented widely on topics related to neurological rehabilitation and to the profession of rehabilitation counseling.

2

THE REHABILITATION EXPERT: ANALYSIS AND MANAGEMENT OF BRAIN INJURY AND OTHER NEUROLOGIC DISORDERS

William H. Burke, Ph.D., CRC

In the last ten years, the role of rehabilitation specialist has developed well beyond the traditional role of rehabilitation counseling and vocational rehabilitation. Rehabilitation specialists today are directly involved in medical and case management from the day of injury through return to work. The rehabilitation specialist is particularly important in catastrophic cases that involve brain injury and other neurologic disorders. In these catastrophic cases, specialized rehabilitation and life care plans are essential to maximize patient function and control long term care costs. Davis (1986) notes that the rehabilitation specialist is actually an extension of the claims department providing expertise in planning and management of the care and controlling costs in these catastrophic cases. He notes that to coordinate services of facilities and professionals, the rehabilitation specialist is best introduced during the acute hospitalization. Working in concert with the claims department, the rehabilitation specialist 1) determines the full extent of the injury, 2) establishes rapport with the claimant, claimant's family, medical facility, claims adjusters and attorneys, 3) assesses the patient's medical and rehabilitation needs, and 4) works in partnership with the claims department to maximize function and contain costs. The goal of the rehabilitation specialist in such claims is to return the injured individual to maximum independence and hopefully the world of work.

Rehabilitation specialists possess unique qualifications that must be carefully assessed prior to developing a consultant relationship. Minimally, the rehabilitation specialist should possess a graduate degree in rehabilitation counseling from a CORE accredited rehabilitation department. The rehabilitation specialist should be board certified by the Commission on Rehabilitation Counselor Certification. He or she should also be actively involved in professional rehabilitation organizations. While many rehabilitation specialists are generalists, it is wise in cases involving a unique population such as those with brain injuries to identify an individual with direct experience treating this population. In addition, when dealing with complex brain injury cases, it is important to seek out an individual with more than merely a passing familiarity with the system of brain injury care and treatment in the United States. And finally, it is critical to ensure the individual has the ability to communicate successfully his or her ideas and plans to third parties. When a qualified rehabilitation specialist is engaged to assist in the planning and management of brain injured patients, reasonable rehabilitation and long term care plans can be formulated and costs can be contained.

The purpose of this chapter is to present a unique and contemporary model of analyzing, planning and managing the brain injury case: Rehabilitation Triage. In an effort to put this method into perspective, the epidemiology, financial considerations and consequences of brain injury will be reviewed followed by an in depth discussion of the process of rehabilitation triage.

Epidemiology

In the last fifteen years, our emergency medical technology, neuroimaging techniques and neurosurgical procedures have improved dramatically resulting in increasing numbers of individuals surviving brain injury each year. Currently the National Head Injury Foundation and the National Institute of Health (1989) estimate that over two million individuals sustain traumatic brain injuries each year. Five-hundred thousand to seven-hundred thousand of these injuries are severe enough to require hospitalization and seventy-five thousand to one-hundred thousand individuals will die each year. However, due to our improved medical technology, the mortality rate has dropped to 5%. Of those who survive brain injury, nearly one-hundred thousand per year will have multiple and permanent physical, cognitive and emotional impairments that will require intensive rehabilitation and often long term care and support. In addition, two-thousand individuals per year will be maintained in a persistent vegetative state (NIH, 1989).

The majority of the brain injured victims are between the ages of fifteen and twenty-five, most are male, and over one-half of all injuries are the result of motor vehicle accidents, followed by falls (21%), assaults and violence (12%), and sports and recreational injuries (10%). No socioeconomic group is spared from this tragic epidemic. The survivors of brain injury come from a variety of educational and vocational backgrounds. However, after brain injury they all will begin a lifelong struggle to live with the residual consequences of their injury. Unlike other acquired disabilities that affect primarily physical function, brain injury can result in persistent cognitive and emotional dysfunction that can compromise community and vocational adjustment. The degree of cognitive and emotional dysfunction will vary from person to person based on the location and severity of the injury to the brain. Until recently, brain injury survivors were frustrating to the rehabilitation profession. Rehabilitation success with brain injured individuals had been considered poor and survivors were often neglected and placed in custodial or psychiatric institutions. Great strides, however, have been made in recent years to compensate for the consequences of brain injury (Burke, Wesolowski & Guth, 1988; Johnston & Lewis, 1991). With appropriate and specialized acute and post-acute or transitional rehabilitation, many brain injured individuals are once again living in the community and are employed. As we all learn more and develop better rehabilitation methods, we can anticipate even greater success in the future (Burke, 1988).

Financial Implications of Brain Injury

The costs of brain injury are staggering. It is estimated that one-hundred-billion dollars in earnings are lost each year as a result of brain injury. $4.5 billion is spent annually to provide medical care and rehabilitation to brain injury survivors. Specialized acute rehabilitation can cost nearly $2,000 per day. Post-hospital transitional rehabilitation costs are in the range of $500-$1000 per day. The ongoing costs of often lifetime care, support and treatment can reach $100,000 per year. It is estimated that the cost to provide care for one brain injured person throughout his or her lifetime can reach 4-5 million dollars (Burke, 1988; Bush, 1990; McMardie & Barker, 1988).

Table 2.1 outlines the cost per year as well as the life expectancy of the five commonly described categories of brain injury (American Re-Insurance, 1993). The costs for the brain injured individual in a deep persistent coma can exceed $200,000, however the life expectancy is generally less that four months. The individual who survives the initial three to four months following a severe injury that remains in a persistent vegetative state constitutes a cost of $185,000 per year for care and treatment with a life expectancy of three to thirty years. The individual who sustains a severe injury, that is with a Glasgow Coma Scale of less than 7, will incur costs of a quarter of a million dollars the year following the injury and lifetime costs are in the range of $32,000 to $100,000 per year. In addition, as noted in Table 2.1, the life expectancy for severe head injured cases at the present time is considered normal. The individual that sustains a moderate injury to the brain, with a Glasgow Coma Scale from 8 to 12, will incur costs of $179,000 in the first year and thereafter cost estimates are $9,000 to $80,000 per year. These individuals are considered to have a normal life expectancy. The significant difference in the range of costs following the first year after a moderate to severe brain injury are largely based on the success of the initial rehabilitation period. If quality and effective rehabilitation are provided to these individuals, the long term, often lifetime costs, can be significantly reduced.

The final category in Table 2.1 notes the mild head injury or the individual with a Glasgow Coma Scale from 13-15. These individuals will have a normal life expectancy; however, this population is so variable the costs cannot be calculated.

The staggering costs of care and treatment following brain injury can, however, be controlled and frequently reduce substantially with 1) comprehensive rehabilitation and life long planning, 2) ongoing management of care and treatment and 3) creative negotiations with rehabilitation providers.

TABLE 2.1 *Estimated Costs of Brain Injury Claims*

Case Category	Cost/Year	Life Expectancy
Deep persistent coma	43,900-208,000	3-4 months
Persistent vegetative state	185,000	3-30 years
Severe	273,750 - year 1; thereafter 32,250-100,000	Normal
Moderate	179,600 - year 1; thereafter 9,000-80,000	Normal
Mild	Varies	Normal

(American Re-Insurance, 1993)

The Consequences of Brain Injury

Brain injury results in a variety of physical, cognitive and emotional impairments that will vary from person to person, depending upon the location of lesion and the severity of the injury. The following discussion will group the deficits following brain injury into four categories (Burke, 1988).

1. *Physical* - Impairments in gait, balance, vision, speech, gross and fine motor control.

2. *Cognitive* - Impairments in attention, memory, information processing, language and conceptualization.

3. *Executive* - Impairments in the ability to plan, organize and executive goal-directed activity and ability to control and regulate behavior.

4. *Behavioral/Emotional* - Impairments that are either the result of the injury to the brain or the individual's psychological reaction to the injury that are manifested in aggression, confusion, disorientation, anxiety, depression and dependence.

Physical Disorders

The physical disabilities are the most obvious and noticeable result of a brain injury. Except with minor head injury, virtually all individuals receiving a traumatic brain injury will experience some initial physical impairment and in some cases, long term physical disability. These physical deficits range from minor disturbances in gross motor function to episodic seizure activity.

Gross motor function is frequently limited by the variances in strength, coordination and the presence of involuntary movement. Each of these areas can range from mild to severe in their impact on an individual's ability to manipulate his environment through body movement. Motor strength can be reduced as in paresis or absent as in plegia. In addition, an increase or decrease in muscle tonus can inhibit the flexibility and coordination of muscle movement. Coordination of complex motor movement can be disrupted as in ataxia by damage to the cerebellum. Other neural damage manifested by coordination disturbance includes position sense or proprioception disturbance. Involuntary movement is disabling simply by its presence, preventing completion of physical tasks. For example, tremor is a term used to describe low intensity rhythmic movement. Spasms or clonis refers to irregular contraction of muscles or muscle groups as seen in some seizure activity.

Visual function is frequently limited by diplopia (double vision) and reduction in the visual field. While generally compensated for, visual disabilities affect all life areas and can raise significant safety concerns. Diplopia may indicate extraoccular muscle weakness. This weakness frequently is a result of cranial nerve damage. Visual field cuts are the result of damage to some portion of the visual pathway. Field cuts can range from total loss of either right or left field to partial loss of each field, depending upon the site of lesion.

Oral motor function can be limited by variances in speech and swallowing. Difficulties in both functions are often related to damage of cranial nerves 9 and 10. Disturbance of the motor component of speech production is referred to as dysarthria. The disturbance ranges from mild to severe depending upon resultant intelligibility. Disturbance of the swallowing function is referred to as dysphagia. As with speech, the level of impairment varies and in extreme cases, the risk of aspiration warrants a mechanism of bypass such as a gastrostomy.

Seizure activity is a frequent consequence of brain trauma. While seizures are categorized into multiple types, all begin with an unusual burst of electrical activity in some area of the brain. Symptoms range from the stereotypical grand mal seizure with total body involvement in changes of consciousness to an absence or focal seizure. The absence or focal seizure is best described as an apparent lapse in concentration or attention. Often these will be the only symptoms. Temporal lobe epilepsy is a relatively recent addition to the categorization of seizure activity. Symptoms are frequently misunderstood, appearing related to emotional and psychological adjustment, rather than manifestations of an organic dysfunction. These symptoms include complex repetitive behaviors and in some cases, unprecipitated rage behaviors. Frequently the individual will have no memory of the actual incident.

Cognitive Disorders

Although the physical disabilities are most obvious following brain injury, the cognitive impairments often are more persistent and debilitating. Cognitive impairments are essentially the result of an alteration in the way information from the environment is perceived, interpreted and processed. Cognitive deficits typically persist throughout one's lifetime and can pose significant barriers to successful community living. The most common cognitive deficits include impairments in attention, judgement, perception, information processing, learning and memory, and communication and language.

Attention is a necessary prerequisite for all other higher mental activities. Our ability to attend to a task or social interaction for a certain period of time while inhibiting our responses to extraneous stimuli allows us to work productively, live independently and maintain social relationships. Many traumatic brain injuries will result in impairments in one's ability to sustain attention, selectively attend to stimuli and shift attention from stimulus to stimulus. The extent of impairment in attention is directly related to the severity of the brain injury.

Many brain injured individuals will suffer impairments in the way they perceive both themselves and their environment. The most problematic impairment in this category is called altered self-perceptions of the brain injured individual. While most brain injured individuals are aware of their physical impairments, they frequently are unaware of their cognitive or emotional deficits. This lack of awareness is often referred to as denial of disability, however it may have a clear neurologic base which is referred to as anosognosia. These individuals don't seem to perceive the extent of their deficits and their effect on returning to pre-morbid lifestyles. Another perceptual problem following brain injury is the misinterpretation of the actions or intentions of other people. These individuals are often described as paranoid, however many merely do not adequately perceive and interpret effective stimuli.

Memory is essentially the process of receiving information, storing it and retrieving it. Most brain injured individuals will complain of memory problems. Impairments in memory are significantly disabling and can persist throughout the individual's lifetime, although improvement is certainly seen with rehabilitation. Brain injured individuals can usually remember their pre-injury life, however frequently cannot recall events immediately prior to their injury. This disorder is referred to retrograde amnesia. Typically the loss of memory prior to the injury can range from 30-60 minutes up to 24 hours. The most disabling memory disorder, however, is the inability to remember new information. This disorder, known as anterograde amnesia, or short term memory, makes it difficult to learn new skills because the individual's ability for immediate recall is impaired. Although improvement can be expected in memory, it is probably more effective to use compensatory strategies than to try to remediate this disorder.

Many brain injured individuals experience a decrease in the speed in which they process information. These individuals react more slowly to stimuli. They also experience slowness in psychomotor activity such as writing and talking. For example, it is not uncommon for the brain injured individual to take 5-10 seconds to respond to a question or to a greeting. This decrease in speed of processing has been found to be related to the individual's perceptual abilities and it also alters problem-solving abilities. This impairment creates great difficulty in social relations and requires patience on the part of families, therapists and co-workers.

A variety of communication and language impairments are seen following brain injury. Unlike the classic language disorders seen with focal brain lesions or strokes, the brain injured survivor will experience more generalized disorders of both receptive and expressive language. These disorders manifest themselves in inefficient word retrieval, difficulty naming objects and reduced word fluency. The individual's expressive communication is impaired because much like an aphasic patient, he or she frequently cannot retrieve the correct word from memory. Other impairments in this area include the individual who simply talks too much. He does not inhibit his communication, thus becoming irritating to people he interacts with. Another language disorder following brain injury is tangential expression of ideas and thoughts. This impairment results in the individual beginning to talk about one subject and then wandering from subject to subject. Although this may be related to selective attention, it is manifested by the individual not being able to focus on one topic but shifting from idea to idea giving others the impression that he is rude or insensitive. This tangential expression is also seen in the individual's writing. Finally, following brain injury the individual may present with the use of peculiar words or phrases. Although this has received little attention in the literature, it has been described as the individual referring to himself in the third person or using peculiar words or phrases in conversation.

Executive Function Disorders

The executive function can be described as the ability to engage in independent, purposeful, self-directed and self-serving behavior. The executive disorders are differentiated from cognitive impairments in the following way: Cognitive impairment implies a specific functional deficit while the executive function affects all aspects of one's life. Deficits in executive functioning are not immediately apparent in casual conversation. Frequently persons with executive function impairments appear cognitively intact. They perform well on neuropsychological examination and when provided with a structured setting, they seem quite normal. Their inability to direct and regulate their behavior, however, seriously interferes with community adjustment. Generally, executive function impairments are manifested by impulsiveness, irritability, rigidity, apathy, carelessness, poor judgement and inappropriate social behavior. These deficits have been described as serious problems in starting, switching and stopping behavior resulting in a decrease in spontaneous behavior, productivity, initiative, and self control, while increasing perseveration, impulsiveness and disinhibition. Executive functions can be conceptualized as consisting of four primary areas: 1) formulating goals, 2) planning and problem-solving, 3) carrying out a plan, and 4) effective performance.

All human activity begins with an intention that is directed toward a goal. If our ability to conceptualize our desires and needs before acting is impaired, the result is impulsive action with little thought of potential consequences or automatic and perseverative responses to stimuli in the environment. The individual with executive function disorders is often unable to formulate goals. It does not occur to the individual to do anything, resulting in an inability to initiate action. Many individuals with executive deficits are capable of performing a task but will not engage in the activity unless directed in a step-by-step manner.

Planning requires an ability to generate alternatives, consider consequences of alternatives, choose an appropriate alternative and develop a framework or road map to direct the activity. In addition, the capacity to sustain attention and to objectively view oneself in the environment is critical to effective planning and problem solving. The inability to initiate a plan is often described as a decrease or absence of motivation and the patient is often referred to as lazy, emotionally disturbed or malingering when in fact the individual lacks the ability to identify the sequential steps to plan the activity. These individuals are often impulsive. When solving problems they act immediately without analyzing options and often the option selected is the same, regardless of the problem at hand. Individuals with planning impairments following brain injury are virtually immobilized by their inability to plan and problem-solve.

Translating an intentional plan into productive or purposeful activity requires the ability to first initiate, switch and stop action in an orderly fashion. Lack of initiative is a frequently complaint of families and is the result of impairments in abstract abilities. The cognitive skills required to carry out complex action are not present. In structured settings, the individual will comply with requests, however will become immobilized when left to self-direction.

To interact successfully with the environment, an individual requires the ability to monitor, self-correct and self-regulate his behavior. Individuals with executive function impairments often do not perceive their mistakes, do not read social cues, and thus do nothing to correct their behavior. They can often discuss their errors but still do nothing to correct behavior. These individuals frequently lack awareness of strengths and deficits resulting in unrealistic self-appraisals. Their deficits in self-awareness also result in their not perceiving errors in performance. They do not pick up on social cues and are unable to be self-critical. These deficits make it difficult for the individuals to profit from their experience. Frequently, individuals will misinterpret social situations, not understand the consequences of their behavior, and misinterpret feedback. This decreased ability to self-regulate behavior often results in socially inappropriate remarks and behavior. This inability to regulate behavior or inhibit impulses is often referred to as disinhibition syndrome. Disinhibited brain injured individuals act before they think. They tell you exactly what they think, are frequently demanding and noncompliant with rules or schedules.

Emotional Behavioral Disorders

Emotional and behavioral disorders pose significant barriers to rehabilitation efforts with the brain injured individual and ultimately these problems can prevent successful community living. Many experts suggest that the emotional and behavior problems are the most difficult to understand, predict and treat of all the consequences of brain injury. The most common emotional/behavioral problems include irritability, agitation, aggression, depression, anxiety, confusion, and denial of deficits.

Although denial can have an organic basis, it is assumed that most brain injured individuals that deny their limitations present with a psychological reaction to their injury. This denial makes rehabilitation efforts difficult. The individual becomes defensive when limitations are pointed out or when realistic goals are discussed. Some individuals will see the rehabilitation setting as the basis for all their problems and actively seek discharge as a solution to these problems. Others will minimize their impairment and when confronted with evidence of limitations such as through therapy, they often become agitated, angry or withdrawn. This denial may be motivated by the need to protect the individual's sense of self. When deficits become more evident and the individual is more aware of limitations, the "catastrophic reaction" will occur, however if progress is not made toward awareness, progress will not be made in rehabilitation.

As disabilities become more evident and the individuals' awareness of limitations increases, it is not uncommon for the brain injured individual to become frustrated, angry, and often depressed. The anger and depression seems most prominent as the individual's denial diminishes. The resulting anger over lost function is naturally directed at family members and therapists. This anger can quickly turn to aggression when the individual will destroy property or strike out in an aggressive way toward family and others. The depression results in withdrawal, social isolation, substance abuse and often suicidal ideation.

Aggression is certainly one of the most troublesome behavior disorders after head injury and several different varieties must be distinguished. In the early stages of recovery, most aggression is caused by confusion and compounded by the alien surroundings of the acute hospital ward. As confusion resolves, the most common problem is one of general irritability which slowly settles over days or months. The most disruptive and distressing form of post-traumatic aggression, especially for families, is the explosive, often dramatic and disruptive, but usually brief outbursts. This typically appears some months after the injury. This disorder has many similarities with epilepsy; delayed onset, paroxysmal, brief duration, dysthymic after effects, and responsiveness to anti-convulsant medication. Although conclusive evidence on its nature is not yet available, it has been referred to a limbic epilepsy. Outbursts may be unprovoked but are more often triggered by trivial frustrations, and curiously, almost never by substantial provocation in much the same way as the reflex epilepsies. Closely related to these aggressive disorders and often associated are intermittent impairments of impulse control and mood changes: sudden depression or hypomanic states which may last for minutes to a few days, beginning and ending as though switched on or off.

Although associated with anger and aggression, the most frequent complaints of families following brain injury are the individual's irritability, impatience, restlessness and agitation. These behaviors may well be the individual's reaction to attempting to do a task that has become quite easy in the past and now is extremely difficult. As the individual's frustration level increases, he becomes more restless and irritable, often resulting in agitated and aggressive behavior. (For a more detailed discussion, the interested reader is referred to Burke, Wesolowski & Blackerby, 1988).

While the consequences of injuries to the brain are varied and complex, significant improvement can be achieved in day-to-day function through appropriate acute and post-acute or transitional rehabilitation. Although brain injury rehabilitation is a new field of study, several myths have emerged that should not be perpetuated. The more prominent myths are presented in this chapter in an effort to dispel these assumptions. (Corthell & Tooman, 1985)

Myths

The first myth has to do with recovery. Most of us experience illness or disease as something that is temporary. Following medical treatment, we will return to our pre-illness functioning. Most victims of brain injury, however, will not completely recover from their trauma and return to pre-injury status. As noted earlier, impairments are typically permanent and can compromise social and vocational functioning. This is not to say that improvement in cognitive, physical and emotional function is not possible. Great improvements can be achieved through rehabilitation. Brain injured victims and their families must understand and accept the limitations that are the result of a brain injury and learn that new life goals may have to be established.

Another myth still perpetuated by many professionals is that whatever recovery or improvement is possible will occur within the first twelve months after the injury to the brain. This one year limit on functional recovery is certainly not true. Research has shown that improvement in functional abilities can be achieved years after even a serious brain injury. It is true that the healing of the brain may occur in the first year but improvement in functional life skills is just beginning. Our present research has demonstrated that significant gains in functional skill development are possible for many years post injury. (Burke, Wesolowski & Guth, 1988; Johnston & Lewis, 1991)

Many families hope that a miracle will happen and their loved one will fully recover and regain all pre-injury abilities. Although this is a normal initial reaction to tragedy, it frequently results in the family changing physicians or rehabilitation programs in hopes that one will produce the miracle. Families that look for this miracle must realize that they are only hindering the rehabilitation process. This myth sets unrealistic expectations for their loved one and reduces the brain injured victim's motivation to actively participate in rehabilitation, thus progress and improvement are slowed. To achieve maximum recovery, rehabilitation is best coordinated by a qualified rehabilitation specialist working in concert with the claims department.

Although many brain injured individuals are labeled as malingerers, the truth is malingering is the exception and not the rule among brain injured victims. Most victims of brain injury are frustrated and want to go on with their lives in a productive fashion. It is true, however, that many brain injured victims learn to depend upon others and develop a "learned helplessness". The learned dependency is the result of others doing so many things for them that they come to believe they are not capable of doing by themselves. The "learned helplessness" (Seligman & Maier, 1967; Seligman, 1990), on the other hand, is the result of repeated failures as the brain injured victim tries to again interact with the environment. At some point, after one more failure, the brain injured individual stops trying all together.

Many brain injured victims report dissatisfaction with their lives, poor social relations, unclear life goals, depression, fear and anxiety. Traditional psychotherapy has not been shown to be the treatment of choice, however. The brain injured victim who participates in traditional psychotherapy often gets worse not better. Their discorded lives are not the result of underlying psychological problems but rather damage to the brain that has produced cognitive and executive deficits. Deficits in attention, memory, problem solving and regulation of social behavior appear to respond more favorably to structured behavior therapeutic strategies.

The myths aside, there are several concerns that truly are related to improvement following brain injury. These include severity of the injury, the victim's pre-injury characteristics, family support, the individuals awareness and acceptance of limitations, the extent and type of rehabilitation, and the long term support in the individual's home community. Brief discussion of these variables related to outcome follows.

It is a common principle that the more severe the injury the less improvement can be expected. Severity is typically measured by length of coma, or length of post-traumatic amnesia. The longer the coma, the more severe the injury. Recent research, however, suggests that while length of coma is related to severity of injury, it appears that the location of the injury is more important than the length of coma. For example, when the frontal lobes of the brain are moderately to severely damaged, regardless of the length of coma, significant deficits in executive function are present. These deficits result in the inability to direct and regulate behavior and significantly interfere with returning to pre-injury lifestyles.

A number of pre-injury variables are also associated with outcome. Those that appear to be most associated with recovery are pre-injury intelligence, cognitive abilities and personality. In developing rehabilitation plans following brain injury, it is critical to analyze these pre-morbid characteristics.

The brain injured victim's family is also critical to improvement in functional abilities. If the family is realistic in its expectations and provides sufficient structure, guidance and support without fostering dependence, the likelihood of improvement is increased. The individual's awareness of limitations and his ability to accept the fact that new life goals often have to be established has also been found to be a critical variable, if not the most important variable associated with successful outcome.

Further, the type and extent of rehabilitation following brain injury has been found to be directly related to improvement in functional abilities. In years past, rehabilitation was discontinued when the individual was medically stable and could be discharged to his home or a nursing home. Later, however, rehabilitation was extended and focused on improving the person's physical abilities, walking and talking. However, today rehabilitation is available to address the wide variety of cognitive, executive and emotional impairment that heretofore prevented independent living and successful return to work.

Another critical variable associated with long term recovery is the support available in the brain injured individual's home community. Many brain injured individuals will require lifelong support to live and work in the community. The extent to which support is available in terms of supported employment, supervised living, brain injury support groups and outreach programs increases the chances of success. In addition, the extent to which government agencies, for example, State Vocational Rehabilitation, Social Security, Mental Health, etc., develop special programs for brain injured individuals greatly increases the chances of long term success.

When considering the above discussion in total, it becomes clear that the brain injury case must be professionally managed. It is critical to analyze pre and post injury function, creatively develop rehabilitation and long term plans of care and manage the ongoing costs of care and treatment. A unique and contemporary approach to the analysis planning and management of the brain injury cases is presented in the following section of this chapter.

Rehabilitation Triage: A Model of Neuro Rehab Management

The "buzz" words today among payors of services for brain injured individuals are "cost containment". However, attempts to contain costs can be short-sighted and actually result in spending far too much on a brain injury claim. With specialized rehabilitation planning, life care planning and ongoing service delivery evaluation, the costs of the brain injury claim can be significantly reduced from the estimated $4-5 million dollars in lifetime medical and care costs. Consider the three cases in Table 2.2. The care and treatment in case #1 was not well planned nor well managed. The carrier involved in this case attempted to contain costs by "curing" the patient rather than developing a realistic and reasonable plan of care, considering the extent and severity of this young man's disabilities. The examples presented in cases #2 and #3 involved comprehensive rehabilitation and life long plans of care. The cost savings in these two cases were substantial yet the patients were provided with rehabilitation to maximize function and long term support was provided to maintain function and prevent decompensation. This process of analyzing the extent of a brain injured individual's disability and developing comprehensive and realistic plans is the basis for the *Rehabilitation Triage* model. The goal of the rehabilitation triage method is to control and reduce the often enormous costs of care and treatment following traumatic brain injury. Rehabilitation triage is a method of comprehensively evaluating the needs of the brain injured survivor and developing a rehabilitation and life care plan that will guide the patient through the rehabilitation maze.

As can be seen in Figure 2.1, the system of medical and rehabilitation following brain injury has become quite sophisticated. In addition, with the significant increase in the number of rehabilitation providers claiming to conduct brain injury rehabilitation, the decision regarding selection of a treatment program must be made carefully. Involving a rehabilitation specialist early on in these cases to conduct this triage approach to cost containment will result in the development of a rehabilitation and life care plan that will establish realistic goals of treatment, provide guidelines to monitor treatment and hold providers accountable for services delivered. (Zasler, 1991) In addition, and most importantly, the rehabilitation specialist can assist the claims department in making the decision when rehabilitation has ended and long term care should begin. This process essentially involves a determination of what type of patient will profit from what type

TABLE 2.2 *Managing Care and Costs*

	No management or coordination of care	Managed and coordinated TBI care	
	Case 1	Case 2	Case 3
Patient	18 year old male TBI GCS=4 coma=6 weeks Disabilities=severe	21 year old male TBI GCS=5 coma=5 weeks Disabilities=severe	17 year old male TBI GCS=5 coma=2 weeks Disabilities= moderate to severe
Acute hospital	246,000	67,200	56,000
Acute rehab	18 months/656,400	7 months/260,400	2 months/76,250
Post acute TBI Rehab	Transitional rehab: 24 months/365,000 Transferred behavioral rehab: 34 months/1,314,000 Transitional: 24 months/401,500	10 months/155,000	6 months/102,300
Psychiatric hospital	260,400	0	0
Long term care	100,375/year (annuity purchased for approximately 1,000,000)	86,870/year (annuity purchased for approximately 870,000)	9,700/year (services included case management, semi-supervised apartment, OT and VOC assistance)
Comments	Patient treated in rehab for 100 months in attempt to find cure	Severe, long term disabilities noted to require life-long supervised care. Rehab goals were to reduce physical and cognitive assistance	(Annuity purchased for approximately 110,000)
Total cost of care and treatment	4,243,300	1,352,600	344,550

of treatment, how long the treatment should continue, and most importantly for cost containment, how to efficiently and cost-effectively meet the long term needs of the moderate to severely brain injured individual.

Rehabilitation triage involves four specific steps:

1. Comprehensive evaluation of the disability;
2. Design of a rehabilitation and life care plan;
3. Selection and negotiation with providers; and
4. Ongoing utilization review and case management.

The goal of this triage method of rehabilitation is not to cure the brain injured patient but to reduce the person's need for physical, cognitive and emotional assistance, which translates into both reduced lifetime costs and a more normal life for the disabled individual. The following is a more detailed outline of the process of rehabilitation triage and life care planning.

Comprehensive Evaluation of Disability

In order to evaluate the merits of a brain injury claim, it is critical to have a comprehensive review of medical records and an analysis of pre-injury function. In addition, and equally important, is an assessment of disabilities or loss of function that can be directly related to the injury to the brain. In order to evaluate the brain injured individual's status prior to the injury, it is important to obtain a number of pre-injury documents. One of the most important documents to discover and one that is too frequently overlooked are the school records of the injured person. An evaluation of school records can assist in identifying the injured individual's pre-morbid intellectual capacity, academic performance and often shed some light on the individual's social and emotional function prior to the injury. In addition, it is important to discover military records, employment records and tax returns. As important as these records are, it is important to discover any and all medical and/or psychiatric

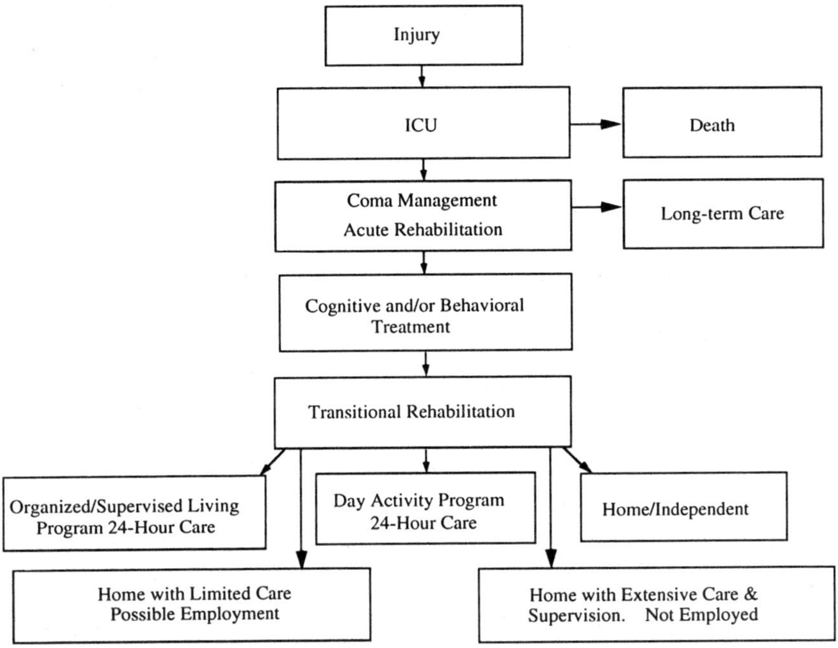

FIGURE 2.1 *Treatment/Care Following Brain Injury*

records that are available prior to the injury. The purpose of this analysis is, of course, to identify any pre-existing conditions, prior injuries and prior medical conditions that relate to the patient's current level of function. In addition, this review will identify current medications whose side effects may include symptoms claimed by the injured person. Following this evaluation of pre-morbid status, it is critical to have a comprehensive evaluation of the patient. The purpose of this evaluation is to establish the individual's level of physical, cognitive and emotional function. In addition, it is often helpful to conduct a vocational assessment to identify transferable work skills and occupations that would be available to the injured individual. This comprehensive evaluation can typically be conducted by a rehabilitation specialist and vocational evaluator. However, in difficult cases, particularly those involving so called minor head injury, it is often necessary to conduct these evaluations in a controlled environment such as a rehabilitation center. Based upon this comprehensive evaluation, if the individual's presentation is considered to be the result of the injury to the brain, the next step in this triage process is to develop a rehabilitation and long term plan of care.

Design of the Rehabilitation and Life Care Plan

When the rehabilitation specialist is working with a brain injured individual that will require aggressive rehabilitation and long term care, it is necessary to have a detailed plan which can provide a guideline for services needed and an estimate of the costs for these services. The rehabilitation and life care plan is designed to provide a clear and effective means of projecting future needs, services and costs in cases involving moderate to severe disability. The method of rehabilitation and life care planning in the triage approach provides a consistent and scientific methodology for assessing the individual's needs and communicating this information clearly to all parties involved. In preparing a rehabilitation and life care plan, the rehabilitation specialist typically serves as a coordinator of interdisciplinary services to provide consistent and quality care for the permanently injured individual. As the coordinator of such services, the rehabilitation specialist is uniquely qualified to develop future life care plans and present such plans to interested parties. This process allows each patient to reach maximum potential regardless of his or her disabilities or vocational interests. The goal of this process is to develop a realistic and cost-effective plan. In order to achieve this goal there are a number of areas which must be considered when establishing the rehabilitation and life care plan. These include the following. (Deutsch & Sawyer, 1985; Deutsch & Fralish, 1991)

1. *Specialized Brain Injury Rehabilitation* - Currently there are over 900 facilities that provide brain injury rehabilitation and the selection of a rehabilitation center must be made

carefully. With appropriate rehabilitation, significant improvements in function can be expected. However, while this specialized rehabilitation can be expensive, it must be viewed as an investment in reducing long term costs of care.

2. *Long Term Care and Treatment* - Following rehabilitation, the catastrophically injured person will require ongoing care and treatment. The primary issue for individuals who require long term care is whether the individual should be placed in a long term care facility or cared for in their home. There is no general answer to this dilemma. A careful analysis of the patient's individual needs and costs of alternatives must be conducted. In addition, a careful analysis of whether skilled (RN or LPN) level care or non-skilled care (aid) must be made. The cost differences are substantial.

3. *Therapeutic Evaluations* - Evaluations are considered separately from therapeutic interventions after rehabilitation as many patients can be provided with daily therapeutic activities by the aids caring for them based on these evaluations. Careful analysis of the patient's potential to benefit from further aggressive therapy can reduce the costs of ongoing care significantly.

4. *Therapy* - Many patients can benefit from ongoing physical, occupational and speech therapy to maintain the gains made during rehabilitation and prevent regression. However, as noted above, the question is whether ongoing therapy must be conducted by licensed therapists. In most cases the answer will be no.

5. *Equipment* - A rehabilitation and long term care plan should outline the patient's ongoing needs for specialized equipment such as wheelchairs, wheelchair accessories, orthopedic equipment, orthotics, etc. In addition, if long term care is provided in the home environment, a variety of

special furnishings and durable medical equipment will be needed, i.e., hospital bed, hoyer lift, suction machine, etc.

6. *Supplies and Medication* - A wide variety of supplies and medications may be required based on the needs of the patient. Future medications for seizures, spasticity, infection, emotional control, etc., must be identified. In addition, supplies such as adult diapers, catheters, feeding supplies, tracheostomy supplies, etc., as well as routine daily supplies must be outlined. In most cases, if long term care is provided in a facility versus home, these supplies are typically included in the negotiated daily facility costs.

7. *Future Medical Care* - Routine medical management is critical to prevent costly medical complications. Routine follow-up by neurology, physiatry, psychiatry, urology, etc., should be clearly outlined in the plan. In addition, anticipated surgical procedures and aggressive medical intervention should be outlined.

8. *Transportation* - The brain injured individual who is wheelchair dependent will require specialized transportation. Typically, a van equipped with a hydraulic lift and chair locks is recommended. However, consideration must be given to the type and cost of a vehicle that the individual would have purchased if not disabled. The cost difference should be outlined in the plan.

9. *Architectural Renovations* - If home care is selected as the most appropriate and cost effective alternative for long term care and treatment, the patient's home often must be modified to accommodate a wheelchair, special furnishings or a live-in attendant. While architectural modifications can be expensive, it must be considered if this one time investment can contain future costs of care.

In addition to maximizing independence and containing future costs, the rehabilitation and life care plan is designed to prevent future costly complications such as skin breakdown, contracture deformities, infection, psychiatric hospitalization, etc.

While considering all the above aspects of a rehabilitation and life care plan, it is important that this plan begin with clear, concise and specific goals of treatment. In addition, the plan should outline decision points that will coordinate movement through the rehabilitation system that was noted in Figure 2.1. The plan should also outline options for long term care and treatment. If appropriately designed, the rehabilitation plan will maximize function which will, in turn, reduce needed services and consequently future costs of care. This planning process must look well beyond the acute care stage of rehabilitation and into the individual's future. There are a wide variety of options for long term support, supervision and care to the catastrophically injured person and, when creatively designed, these can typically be conducted in the community quite reasonably.

It should also be noted that a large number of individuals are currently involved in developing rehabilitation and long term plans of care. It is often necessary to engage a rehabilitation specialist with particular expertise in the area of brain injury to review and analyze rehabilitation and life care plans that are produced by others. The purpose of this analysis and review is to evaluate these plans for their accuracy, merit and cost effectiveness.

Case Management and Utilization Review

As we have seen up to this point, brain injury rehabilitation can be long, complex, and enormously expensive. Coile (1994) notes that "case management of rehabilitation patients will become almost universal within the next five years" (p. 62). However, specialized case management and supervision of brain injury rehabilitation and long term care services is essential to ensure quality of services, evaluate appropriateness of treatment being delivered, and to determine when rehabilitation is over and long term support should begin.

The critical variable in this aspect of the rehabilitation triage process is to identify the most appropriate provider for each level of care. Ten years ago only a handful of treatment facilities existed in the United States that were dedicated to brain injury rehabilitation and virtually no specialized facilities existed to provide long term support and supervision. Today, over 900 facilities are operating in the United States that claim to have special expertise in the rehabilitation and long term care of brain injured individuals. It is estimated that brain injury rehabilitation has become a 4 billion dollar industry (Cope & O'Lear, 1993). However, while these facilities have opened at a rapid rate over the past several years, the development of professional expertise as well as treatment strategies for this special population have not kept pace with the program openings. Ashley and Krych (1990), point out that there is currently a lack of wide spread expertise in the treatment of brain injured patients. They further note that significant variability exists in terms of service delivery models, treatment effectiveness and treatment outcomes. As noted earlier, specialized brain injury rehabilitation represents a significant expense; however, if successful, this investment can maximize patient function and significantly reduce long term care costs. It is therefore critical to both the patient and the payor to seek guidance from a rehabilitation specialist not only with expertise with this special population, but who also understands the brain injury rehabilitation system in the United States. The rehabilitation specialist can work in concert with the payor to identify the most appropriate and clinically relevant treatment program as well as evaluate the care and treatment over time.

Another aspect of the rehabilitation specialist's role in this area of case management and utilization review is to negotiate costs of services with providers and establish time frames for renegotiation. As noted above, the costs of rehabilitation and long term care can be staggering; however, these costs can be managed with creative negotiating by a rehabilitation specialist familiar with the brain injury rehabilitation system. Moreover, costs can be managed if the case is well monitored and a clinical determination is made regarding when aggressive rehabilitation should be discontinued.

Currently, no objective measure is available to make this determination, and until such a measure is developed, families and payors must rely on the often contradictory subjective clinical advise of treating therapists. A rehabilitation specialist with specialized expertise with brain injured individuals can serve as the team leader and more objectively identify progress and generate concensus regarding the decision to continue or discontinue aggressive therapy.

When the decision has been made to transition the patient from active rehabilitation to long term supported, supervised placement, ongoing specialized case management is needed to maintain the brain injured individual's level of function achieved during rehabilitation and prevent medical complications and emotional and/or functional regression. Through ongoing evaluation and monitoring of patient care, appropriate levels of care and treatment can be maintained and problems prevented. With the limited number of rehabilitation specialists with particular expertise in brain injury, this ongoing management is best performed by assigning a medical or rehabilitation case manager to the case for day-to-day management and utilizing the rehabilitation specialist as a consultant to these day-to-day case managers.

Rehabilitation triage is a comprehensive and efficient method of controlling costs by utilizing experts in the area of brain injury to assist with claims management. In the worst case scenario with expert brain injury rehabilitation planning and management, the $4-$5 million in estimated life time costs can be substantially reduced. The outcome of this rehabilitation triage method is:

1. Creative cost-effective plans of care that can significantly control damages;
2. Insures quality of care;
3. Avoids duplication of services;
4. Plans are designed to maximize function;
5. Identifies transferable work skills; and
6. Provides a detailed outline of future care needs.

Case Examples

In an effort to bring the process of rehabilitation triage to life, following are two case examples. The first case involves a traumatic brain injury. The second case describes a gentleman who suffered from an electric shock.

Case 1: Scott

Scott is a forty-three year old man who sustained a traumatic brain injury secondary to a motor vehicle accident. He was found unresponsive at the scene of the accident and was transported by ambulance to the local emergency room. On arrival at the E.R. he continued to present as unresponsive with a Glasgow Coma Scale of 6. Initial CT-scan of the brain revealed right cerebral contusions. Scott remained in a comatose condition for approximately thirteen days. His neurologic condition gradually improved and he was transferred to acute rehabilitation. He participated in a hospital-based rehabilitation program for two weeks. He was discharged to his home in the care of his wife with arrangements for outpatient occupational therapy. He participated in outpatient occupational therapy two times per week for approximately four months. Physically, Scott improved significantly during rehabilitation, however he continued to present with cognitive and behavioral impairments secondary to his traumatic brain injury. Prior to this motor vehicle accident, Scott was in good health with no history of severe illness or injury. He was married with no children. He was a college graduate employed in a professional capacity. Scott was referred by his insurance case manager for evaluation of his current status and recommendations for further treatment.

On evaluation, Scott presented with no obvious physical disabilities. He presented with some left-sided weakness; however, this did not interfere with his day-to-day function. Cognitively, Scott presented with impairments of attention and memory. His memory for immediate, recent and remote information was significantly impaired. His expressive language was fluent; however, he presented with moderate word finding difficulties. In addition, his language was often tangential and perseverative. He often appeared confused during evaluation. Behaviorally, Scott presented rather childlike and dependent. His behavior was impulsive and he was often socially inappropriate. Scott also presented with impairments of overall executive function. He presented with moderate to severe impairments of problem solving, planning, and overall abstract abilities. His thought processes were quite concrete. Scott was generally independent in self-care; however, he required cues to maintain appropriate hygiene.

At the time of this evaluation, Scott was living with his wife in a modest, three-bedroom home. His wife was employed in a professional capacity in the public relations industry. Scott had not returned to work since the time of his motor vehicle accident and generally spent his time unproductively in the home watching television. All rehabilitation efforts had been discontinued.

Based on this evaluation, it was clear that Scott had received only limited rehabilitation and the intervention was focused primarily on his physical recovery. His wife was becoming quite frustrated with her new role of caretaker and while she did state that she wanted to maintain their relationship, she felt that she could not continue the relationship with Scott's present condition. A rehabilitation plan was developed to provide Scott with specialized brain injury rehabilitation in his home and surrounding community. As a result of his cognitive and behavioral disabilities, he was not a candidate to return to work. The goals of this rehabilitation effort were to improve his independence in self-care and activities of daily living, assist him in compensating for his memory impairment, improve his social skills, and develop a daily structured routine that would include a daily productive avocational activity.

A rehabilitation psychologist was recruited from a nearby university to coordinate the implementation of this rehabilitation plan. In cooperation with this psychologist, an occupational therapist and cognitive therapist were recruited to conduct the therapeutic portion of his in-home rehabilitation program. Undergraduate students at the local university were recruited to serve as personal care attendants to teach Scott household management and avocational activities. A computer and printer were also introduced as cognitive orthotics. When the rehabilitation team was organized, the plan was implemented over a four-month period. At the end of the four months, Scott's rehabilitation was concluded. His computer was loaded with daily to-do lists, task analyses of household tasks, instructions for routine activities, etc. His daily routine included four hours making wood products in his garage which was a hobby in which he engaged prior to the motor vehicle accident. In an effort to insure continuation of his daily routine and prevent complications, he was provided with the ongoing assistance of a personal care assistant five hours per day, Monday through Friday. The rehabilitation psychologist who coordinated this initial rehabilitation effort was contracted to provide follow-up evaluations and in an effort to provide guidance to the personal care attendants. These evaluations were conducted semi-annually during the first year and thereafter on an annual basis. Individual counseling was arranged for Scott's wife to ensure that she was provided with the support necessary to maintain her relationship with Scott. A case manager was also recruited to provide overall supervision and guidance of the ongoing care as well as to recruit, hire, train and supervise the personal care attendant.

The rehabilitation program that was conducted in Scott's home was very successful in restructuring his daily activities, compensating for his cognitive impairments, and improving his social skills. At the present time, three years after implementation of this plan, Scott continues to live with his wife. He has become essentially a house-husband and with the assistance of his personal care attendant and computer, he adequately maintains the home, does all the cooking, and works in his woodshop four to five hours per day. It should be noted that the alternative for Scott if his wife were no longer available to provide assistance and supervision was placement of Scott in a supervised living center or providing him with live-in care as well as daily personal care assistance. In either case, the costs are significantly greater than the results of this community rehabilitation and long term care program.

Following is an outline of the costs associated with his rehabilitation and lifelong care plan.

TABLE 2.3 *Rehabilitation and Life Care Plan*

Specialized Rehabilitation:

Recommendation	Frequency/Duration	Cost
Intensive Community Rehabilitation	6 hours/day for 4 months only	$21,600
Occupational Therapist	1-2 hours/day during rehabilitation only	N/A: Included in 21,600 rehabilitation costs
Speech/Cognitive Therapist	1-2 hours/day during rehabilitation only	N/A: Included in 21,600 rehabilitation costs
Personal Care Assistant	6 hours/day	N/A: Included in 21,600 rehabilitation costs
Rehabilitation Psychologist/ Team Leader	4 hours/week for 1 month; then 2 hours/week for 3 months only	3,400 (Based on 85/hour)
	Total Cost of Rehabilitation:	**25,000**

Therapeutic Evaluations/Therapy:

Recommendation	Frequency/Duration	Cost
Rehabilitation Psychologist	2 times/year for 1 year following rehabilitation; then annually	340 the first year; then 170/year (Based on 85/hour x 2 hours/ evaluation)
Personal Care Assistant (PCA)	5 hours/day, Monday-Friday to Life Expectancy	10,400/year (Based on 8/hour)
Miscellaneous Costs of PCA (FICA, Accounting, Payroll, etc.)	N/A	1,560/year (Based on 15% of payroll)

Continued

TABLE 2.3 *Rehabilitation and Life Care Plan, continued*

Therapeutic Evaluations/Therapy:

Recommendation	Frequency/Duration	Cost
Counseling for Scott's Wife	1 time/week for 6 months; then 2 times/month	3,060 the first year; then 2,040/year (Based on 85/session)
Case Manager	4 hours/month	2,880/year (Based on 60/hour)

Equipment/Supplies:

Recommendation	Frequency/Duration	Cost
Macintosh Computer with Color Monitor and Printer	1 time/5 years	1,896
Compatible Software	Annually	800 the first year; then 300/year

The cost during the first year of this intervention, which included the intensive community rehabilitation program, was $40,989. From year two through Scott's life expectancy, the annual cost is approximately $17,729 per year. This represents a cost of $1,477 per month or $48.57 per day to maintain Scott in the community.

Case 2: John

John is a fifty-two year old man who was injured secondary to an electric shock. He was rendered unconscious and suffered serious burns. He was transported to the local emergency room by ambulance where he was stabilized and transferred by air to the regional medical center burn unit. When John arrived at the burn unit he presented as paralyzed with second and third degree burns on his face, arms and hands. He was treated at the burn center for seven weeks. In addition to his burns, he also was diagnosed with a T-5 compression fracture, neurogenic pain, and closed head injury. Following his stabilization at the burn unit, John was transferred to a rehabilitation hospital in his home community. On admission he presented as quadriparetic. His cognitive function appeared within normal limits. The goals of his rehabilitation program were to improve his mobility, increase his independence in self-care, and increase his strength and endurance. He remained an inpatient for five months at the rehabilitation hospital. At that time he was discharged to the care of his wife with continued outpatient therapy arranged Monday through Friday, three hours per day. He was also provided with a personal care assistant in his home sixteen hours per day.

John was referred by the Workers Compensation carrier for comprehensive evaluation of his disabilities, evaluation of his current care and treatment program, as well as recommendations for future care and treatment.

John presented for evaluation as alert, oriented, and generally cooperative. He presented in a power wheelchair; however, with prompting he was able to ambulate 500 feet with the aid of a walker, although his balance was mildly impaired. He was independent in all transfers to and from his wheelchair. John presented with full range of motion throughout. His upper extremity grasp and fine motor function were within normal limits on the right; however, fine motor function was impaired on the left. His overall physical endurance and stamina were decreased and he had gained fifty pounds since his accident. He required minimum assistance with self-care and activities of daily living, but at the time of this evaluation he is being provided with total assistance by his personal care attendant and his wife. Cognitively, John complained of impaired memory, although on examination his overall cognitive function was within functional limits for day-to-day living. Emotionally, he presented as quite stable and was motivated to increase his independence. However, he believed he was dependent on others and that he was severely disabled.

Based upon this evaluation and analysis of his current treatment program, a rehabilitation plan was developed. The goals of this plan were to increase his physical abilities for household ambulation, increase his independence in self-care and activities of daily living, and change his perception from one of dependent to independent. Due to his injuries, age and education, return to work was not considered a potential outcome and during the period of recommended rehabilitation, daily routines and activities would be developed to create a lifestyle similar to that of a retired person. The rehabilitation plan recommended a four month period of inpatient post-hospital rehabilitation. The outcome of this rehabilitation program was to increase his ability to ambulate short distances and certainly to become a household ambulator, increase his upper extremity strength and fine motor function, identify adaptive equipment to compensate for his impaired bimanual function, and decrease his weight by 40-50 pounds. Following this rehabilitation program, John's needs for daily personal care attendant services were reduced from 16 to 4-6 hours per day. The personal care attendant services following rehabilitation were designed to provide John with the assistance he needed, yet to foster a sense of independence. In addition, following rehabilitation, physical and occupational therapy evaluations were recommended to maintain his level of function. Based upon these evaluations, daily therapeutic activities were conducted by his personal care attendants. Ongoing medical follow-up and accident-related medications were also included in his long term plan.

The cost of John's treatment and daily care at the time of this evaluation was $79,680 per year. After implementation of this rehabilitation plan and an initial investment of $48,000 in specialized inpatient rehabilitation, the annual costs of John's care and treatment were reduced to $19,366 per year. This reduction of $60,314 per year represents a savings over his anticipated life expectancy of over 1.2 million dollars. In addition to the financial savings, John's life following the development and implementation of this plan is certainly more meaningful and he is more independent. John presently enjoys a retirement lifestyle and no longer perceives himself as dependent.

References

Ashley M.J. & Krych, D.K. (1990). Considerations on the purchase of post acute rehabilitation services. *Journal of Insurance Medicine.* 22(3), 230-234.

Burke, W.H. (1988). *Head Injury Rehabilitation: An Overview.* Houston, TX: HDI Publishers (2nd Edition in press).

Burke, W.H., Wesolowski, M.D. & Blackerby, W. (Eds.). (1988). *Rehabilitation and Treatment of Traumatic Brain Injury.* Houston, TX: HDI Publishers (2nd Edition in press).

Burke, W.H., Wesolowski, M.D., & Guth, M. (1988). Comprehensive head injury rehabilitation: An outcome evaluation. *Brain Injury,* 2, 313-322.

Bush, G.W. (1990). Calculating the cost of long term services: A four-step process. *Journal of Head Trauma Rehabilitation.* 5(1), 47-56.

Coile, R.C. (1994). Forecasting the future: The top 10 trends for rehabilitation in the 1990's. *Rehab Management,* Feb/March, 59-63.

Cope, D.N. & O'Lead, J. (1993). A clinical and economic perspective on head injury rehabilitation. *Journal of Head Trauma Rehabilitation,* 8(4), 1-14.

Corthell, D.W. & Tooman, M. (1985). *Twelfth Institute on Rehabilitation Issues: Rehabilitation of TBI.* Menomonie, WI: University of Wisconsin, Stout.

Davis, W.W. (1986). Managing the brain injured insurance case. *Trends in Rehabilitation,* 13-17.

Deutsch, P.M. (1989). Discharge planning: Structuring the home environment. In Deutsch, P.M. & Fralish, K. (Eds). *Innovations in Head Injury Rehabilitation.* New York, NY: Mathew Bender.

Deutsch, P.M. & Sawyer, H.W. (1985). *A Guide to Rehabilitation.* New York, NY: Mathew Bender.

Guidelines for Reserving: Traumatic Brain Injury (1993). Princeton, NJ: American Re-Insurance Company.

Johnston, M. & Lewis, F. (1991). Outcomes of community re-entry programs for brain injured survivors. *Brain Injury,* 5, 141-154.

Interagency Head Injury Task Force Report (1989). National Institute of Neurologic Disorders and Stroke. Bethesda, MD: National Institute of Health.

McMardie, W.R. & Barker, S.L. (1988). The financial trauma of head injury. *Brain Injury,* 2(4), 357-364.

Seligman, M. & Maier, S. (1967). Failure to escape traumatic shock. *Journal of Experimental Psychology,* 74, 1-9.

Seligman, M. (1990). *Learned Optimism.* New York, NY: Pocket Books.

Zasler, N.D. (1992). Neuromedical advances in traumatic brain injury rehabilitation care. *The Neurolaw Letter*, 2(3).

William H. Burke, Ph.D., CRC

Dr. Burke is recognized internationally for his expertise in the field of brain injury. He designed three of the earliest brain injury rehabilitation centers in the U.S. and today he consults with rehabilitation centers, attorneys, insurance companies and governmental agencies throughout the U.S. and Canada. He is a well known author in the field of brain injury rehabilitation and lectures on the topic nationally. Dr. Burke is currently completing the manuscript of a text book entitled *Critical Pathways in Neurologic Rehabilitation.*

3

CASE ANALYSIS IN FORENSIC REHABILITATION: A MULTIAXIAL APPROACH

David R. Price, Ph.D.

The first step in the determination of the reasonableness and need for any rehabilitation care plans in forensic settings is to determine the validity of the claim. In cases of simple physical injury this is relatively straight forward. However, in claims of head injury or psychological trauma secondary to physical injury the task becomes very complex given the often subjective, self reported symptoms. To determine the validity of a claim, the claims executive will need to identify whether an injury or deficit secondary to a cause of action has occurred or not. To determine whether an injury is post-cause of action, the claims or case manager will need to assess the functioning of the individual pre- and post-cause of action.

Claims Analysis

The evaluation of the claimant post cause of action will typically include appropriate independent medical evaluations by appropriate specialists, who should be able to determine the current level of functioning of the litigant. Unfortunately this will always occur after an alleged cause of action and the examiner often mistakenly attributes all symptoms, including those that were pre-existing, to the traumatic event that is the focus of the litigation or claim.

After an injury has occurred, and if liability has been assumed or assigned, the claims executive will need to determine the extent of the injury and the validity of the settlement or rehabilitation costs. The traditional settlement demand will include demands for hedonistic damages, reimbursement for pain and suffering, lost income, and the cost for rehabilitation and aftercare. In the absence of substantial physical findings and documentation (i.e., positive CT Scan, MRI, X Rays etc.) this task becomes monumental.

Assuming the claims executive has decided the claim for damages is legitimate, the next task requires the determination of the appropriateness and need for reimbursement and/or rehabilitation of the alleged losses and/or symptoms claimed. The determination of the reasonableness of claimed losses for hedonistic damages and lost income is beyond the scope of this chapter. This chapter will address the determination of the reasonableness and need for the rehabilitation and aftercare plans in cases where liability has been assumed.

Rehabilitation Plan Analysis

The analysis of rehabilitation and treatment plans often involves two stages. The first stage is to determine the validity and severity of the injury claimed. The second stage should focus on identifying the areas of the rehabilitation plans that need to be retained or increased, the areas of rehabilitation that are wasteful or unnecessary, and the areas for which no liability should be assumed.

In cases of physical injuries that include claims of psychological injury it is extremely difficult to determine the validity of the claimed psychological symptoms, given their often subjective nature. Often these are simply subjective self reports by the claimant that there has been a loss of memory, attention and/or concentration ability, motivation, and cognitive skill. These can only be addressed if the claimant has been properly evaluated and diagnosed. Traditional diagnoses such as Postconcussional Syndrome, Post-traumatic Stress Disorder, or Reactive Depression are of little utility to the claims executive. They do not address specific deficits and are of little value in rehabilitation planning since not only do they not address rehabilitation needs, they also do not differentiate between pre-existing and post-injury conditions nor do they tease out concurrent mental or physical conditions for which no liability is assumed. Consequently, such descriptive diagnoses only serve to confuse the claims executive by attributing any and all emotional, cognitive and behavioral symptoms and deficits to one incident specific condition when there could be multiple factors of causation for which the insurer would not be liable. This approach is reductionistic and overly simplistic. When using such a simplistic approach, clinicians tend to look at only a narrow band of the client's behavior and symptoms and make incomplete and incorrect judgments regarding diagnosis, rehabilitation and treatment.

Mental health professionals abandoned this simplistic approach in the past and replaced it with a comprehensive "multiaxial" approach to diagnosis. This approach attempts to consider the full range of mental, emotional, physical, and psychosocial factors that can produce psychopathology, cognitive impairment, and psychiatric conditions. This multiaxial approach focuses on the identification of all conditions, both pre-existing and post traumatic, that can produce mental, emotional or cognitive symptoms or deficits. This approach can be extremely useful in forensic settings (Price & Price, 1992).

The Multiaxial Analysis

Pages 8-31 of the Diagnostic and Statistical Manual of Mental Disorders-Third Edition [DSM-III]; pages 15-21 of its revision [DSM-III-R]; and pages 25-34 of the new Diagnostic and Statistical Manual of Mental Disorders-Fourth Edition [DSM-IV], published by the American Psychiatric Association, outline a five part diagnostic system to be used in evaluating patients. This multiaxial system contains five areas that clinicians must examine to fully understand, diagnose and treat their patients. Without the use of these guidelines, clinicians tend to misdiagnose, under diagnose, or otherwise misinterpret their client's symptoms and behavior.

This multiaxial approach is extremely useful in forensic rehabilitation. When carefully applied this diagnostic system will aid in identifying any and all clinical syndromes present. These can range from a possible Post-traumatic Stress Disorder related to the trauma that is a focus of litigation to the identification of a pre-existing condition such as Dementia associated with alcoholism, that would not be compensable. The utility and application of each individual axis to forensic rehabilitation will be discussed below.

Axis I

The first axis of the multiaxial system is Axis I, where Clinical and Organic Syndromes are identified. This diagnostic category includes over 200 mental disorders. Diagnosis of each mental disorder requires the observance or history of specific symptoms. Because most patients present with mixed symptoms, multiple Axis I diagnoses may be made. Relative to head injuries, which are found in many forensic rehabilitation cases, one may find a diagnosis such as Organic Personality Disorder (DSM-III-R 310.10) or Personality Change Due To A General Medical Condition (DSM-IV 310.1) on Axis I. Knowledge of this diagnosis would allow the claims executive to refer to the DSM-III-R or to DSM-IV and find an objective description of the condition.

One may also find on this axis other disorders relative to rehabilitation which could contribute to reported cognitive or psychological symptoms and be pre-existing, thus, arguably noncompensable. This would include such conditions as Alcohol Dependence (DSM-III-R 303.90; DSM-IV 303.9), Sedative, Hypnotic Or Anxiolytic Dependence (DSM-III-R 304.10; DSM-IV 304.10), Hypochondriasis (DSM-III-R 300.70; DSM-IV 300.7), Attention-Deficit Hyperactivity Disorder (DSM-III-R 314.01; DSM-IV 314.01), Malingering (DSM-III-R V65.20; DSM-IV V65.20)), or Marital Problem (DSM-III-R V61.10) which is known as a Partner Relational Problem (DSM-IV V61.1) in DSM-IV.

Often in litigation the actual physical injury is associated with a psychological injury in order to target the policy limit in the claims for damages. This is not to say that psychological injury does not occur simultaneously with physical insult, but that it is often misdiagnosed or improperly assessed. Depression, which is often claimed in forensic cases, is a symptom, not a disorder. If one peruses DSM-III-R or DSM-IV one would find that depression is a possible symptom in over 200 diagnosable conditions. Anxiety, also often claimed in litigated cases, is also a symptom and not a disorder. Anxiety, which is caused by many sources, is also a symptom in over 200 diagnosable conditions in DSM-III-R and DSM-IV. Since research estimates that the prevalence rate is 28.1% of the adult population for the occurrence of a mental or addictive disorder (Regier, Narrow, Rae, Manderscheid, Locke, & Goodwin, 1993) there is a reasonable probability that a plaintiff or litigant had one or more pre-existing mental or addictive disorder whose treatment and/or rehabilitation will need to be addressed by a rehabilitation plan but whose cost of care would not, or should not, be reimbursable by a defendant. The comprehensive rehabilitation plan in forensic settings will address these issues and tease their cost out of the overall plan.

It is crucial to the defendant or insurer in forensic rehabilitation to identify any symptoms that are consciously produced, whether they be physical or psychological. There is an index of suspicion found in DSM-III, DSM-III-R, and DSM-IV that suggests when to suspect malingering (See Chapter 11 on malingering). The first item in this index is "medicolegal context of presentation." This would mean that any rehabilitation plan should consider and rule out the presence of malingering in the litigant. Malingering is the conscious production of symptoms for ulterior gain. Symptoms may be consciously produced in Factitious disorders as well. In those cases the symptoms are produced in order to assume the role of the patient. Should the presence of either of these disorders be identified in the rehabilitation plan, the insurer should be aware that the disorder, and the symptoms produced within it, are not compensable.

Physical and psychological symptoms may also be unconsciously produced. The identification of a condition such as Body dysmorphic disorder, Conversion disorder, Hypochondriasis, Somatization disorder, Somatoform pain disorder, or

Undifferentiated somatoform disorder should alert the rehabilitation advisor and/or insurer that a condition is present that produces symptoms that have no clear pathophysiologic process and in which psychological factors are felt to be etiologically related to the symptoms. These disorders are arguably compensable and should always be challenged by the defendant.

Substance abuse disorders are also diagnosed on this axis. While this is frequently an area that is ignored in many rehabilitation plans, it should never be ignored in forensic settings. Physical or psychological symptoms secondary to pre-existing or current substance abuse are not typically compensable rehabilitation issues. Abused substances can be of a recreational drug type (alcohol, cannabis, inhalants) or a prescribed medication (pain killer, sedative, anti-anxiety). The abuse of drugs, whether prescribed or recreational, can produce symptoms which include loss of libido, emotional lability, dementia, liver damage, loss of concentration and/or depression.

Organic disorders are also found on Axis I. Often the diagnosed organic disorder will be a focus of litigation and rehabilitation, as in head injury claims. These conditions may have other, noncompensable causes as well that may be diagnosed on Axis III. There are 213 diagnosable conditions in DSM-III-R that may produce symptoms such as memory impairment, concentration problems, confusion or slow reaction times that may be mistakenly attributed to a compensable organic condition that is related to a case of action by a plaintiff or his/her expert. Noncompensable organic conditions would be those related to substance abuse or etiology unrelated to the cause of action. These could range from pre-existing head injury to Progressive supranuclear palsy, Cranial arteritis, Arteriovenous malformation, Cerebral embolism, Metabolic, endocrine, and nutritional disorders or Hepatic, renal, or pulmonary failure. Dementia is an organic disorder often diagnosed on this axis. Dementia is the loss of acquired intelligence as opposed to retardation, which is the failure to acquire intelligence. Any organic diagnosis needs to have its etiology carefully identified for appropriate assignation of compensability and treatment.

Pre-existing disorders are of special interest in forensic rehabilitation since they exist prior to the cause of action and the defendant would have no liability for their remediation. Often neglected in the rehabilitation plan is the documentation of disorders that arise in childhood or adolescence, which would normally predate the cause of action. Disorders of note that occur in childhood and that can cloud plaintiffs' symptoms and theories of casualty include Attention deficit hyperactivity disorders, Bulimia nervosa, and Anorexia nervosa. These disorders can be particularly troubling in rehabilitation plans for head injured litigants. Attention deficit hyperactivity disorders have symptoms of poor attention span, concentration difficulties, and poor neurometric test performance. They often produce symptoms claimed to be the result of closed head injury. Equally troubling are disorders of appetite such as bulimia and anorexia which can be life threatening, produce EEG changes, and coexist with mood disorders. The existence of these disorders needs to be documented in the pre-existing medical, pediatric, dental or psychological records.

The comprehensive forensic rehabilitation plan includes the identification of conditions that may be a focus of mental health intervention, but are not mental disorders in and of themselves. In DSM-III and DSM-III-R these are called V codes and are used to identify things such as marital problems, parent-child problems, and occupational problems, to name a few. In cases of catastrophic injury such as traumatic brain damage or spinal cord paralysis these events may be secondary to the cause of action. They may also be pre-existing conditions which need to be identified by proper evaluation and discovery.

There may exist incident specific conditions secondary to the cause of action that need to be addressed in the rehabilitation plans. Because these conditions would be a consequence of the cause of action they would likely be compensable. The most likely claimed condition is the Post-traumatic stress disorder. While emotionally distressing it is usually not totally disabling. Less severe emotional reactions would be Adjustment Disorders that remit within 6 months of onset and the Acute stress reaction which will be included in

DSM-IV. These conditions which are less severe than PTSD need to be identified as they will effect the overall rehabilitation cost estimate included in the rehab plan.

Axis II

The second axis, or Axis II, found in the multiaxial system contains disorders that are considered to be developmental in nature, such as personality disorders or developmental delays. Personality disorders are felt to be in existence by late adolescence and likely predate the cause of action. There are 12 pathological types of personalities. Many plaintiffs frequently have definite, Axis II personality disorders that pre-exist the cause of action. It may be that the personality disorder characteristics are the basis of the claim or litigation. For example, plaintiffs with an Antisocial Personality Disorder may be diagnosed with Frontal Lobe Syndrome when their symptoms are actually the result of their personality disorder and not their alleged head injury. Plaintiffs' psychological and psychiatric expert witnesses rarely diagnose or admit the existence of these non proximate conditions because such an admission would cloud their Axis I diagnosis.

Overall, Personality disorders often go unrecognized by treatment providers, examiners and rehabilitation experts. Personality disorders usually will predate the cause of action and not be compensable. More importantly, personality disorders predispose individuals to other mental disorders which the defendant would arguably not be liable for. Price (1994) reports the following personality disorders and their often coexisting or related conditions that the rehabilitation expert needs to be alert for:

Paranoid Personality Disorder

Frequent Co-existing Conditions:

- Schizophrenia
- Delusional (Paranoid) Disorder
- Brief Reactive Psychosis

Schizoid Personality Disorder

Frequent Co-existing Conditions:

Schizophrenia

Brief Reactive Psychosis

Possible Co-existing Personality Disorders:

Borderline Personality Disorder

Schizotypal Personality Disorder

Frequent Co-existing Conditions:

Schizophrenia

Brief Reactive Psychosis

Major Depression

Possible Co-existing Personality Disorders:

Borderline Personality Disorder

Antisocial Personality Disorder

Predisposing Conditions:

Attention-Deficit Hyperactivity Disorder

Conduct Disorder

Frequent Co-existing Conditions:

Somatization Disorder

Pathological Gambling

Psychoactive Substance Abuse Disorder (including but not limited to alcohol abuse/dependence)

Malingering

Borderline Personality Disorder

Predisposing Conditions:

Bulimia Nervosa

Identity Disorder

Frequent Co-existing Conditions:

Schizophrenia

Brief Reactive Psychosis

Dysthymia

Multiple Personality Disorder

Trichotillomania

Major Depression
Psychoactive Substance Abuse (including but not limited to alcohol abuse/dependence)
Bipolar Disorder

Possible Co-existing Personality Disorders:

Schizotypal Personality Disorder
Histrionic Personality Disorder
Narcissistic Personality Disorder
Antisocial Personality Disorder

Histrionic Personality Disorder

Frequent Co-existing Conditions:

Brief Reactive Psychosis
Dysthymia
Conversion Disorder
Somatization Disorder

Narcissistic Personality Disorder

Frequent Co-existing Conditions:

Brief Reactive Psychosis
Dysthymia
Major Depression
Psychoactive Substance Abuse (including but not limited to alcohol abuse/dependence)

Possible Co-existing Personality Disorders:

Histrionic Personality Disorder
Borderline Personality Disorder
Antisocial Personality Disorder

Avoidant Personality Disorder

Predisposing Conditions:

Avoidant Disorder of Childhood or Adolescence

Frequent Co-existing Conditions:

Delusional Disorder
Dysthymia
Agoraphobia without history of Panic Disorder
Social phobia

Dependent Personality Disorder

Predisposing Conditions:

Chronic physical illness in childhood or adolescence
Separation Anxiety Disorder in childhood or adolescence

Frequent Co-existing Conditions:

Dysthymia
Conversion Disorder
Major Depression

Obsessive Compulsive Personality Disorder

Frequent Co-existing Conditions:

Obsessive Compulsive Disorder
Hypochondriasis
Major Depression
Dysthymia

Passive Aggressive Personality Disorder (Recognized in DSM-III-R but not in DSM-IV)

Frequent Co-existing Conditions:

Major Depression
Dysthymia
Alcohol Abuse/Dependence

Of equal concern in determining rehabilitation needs following closed head injuries is the presence of Developmental disorders, which are diagnosed on Axis II under DSM-III-R guidelines but will be diagnosed under Axis I in DSM-IV as a "disorder usually first diagnosed in Infancy, Childhood, or Adolescence". These are disorders that have significant implications in all head injury claims and seldom receive their due attention. Developmental disorders include learning disabilities such as Developmental Reading Disorder (DSM-III-R 315.00), Developmental Receptive Language Disorder (DSM-III-R 315.31), and Developmental Coordination Disorder (DSM-III-R 315.40). Examples of these disorders in DSM-IV (which would be listed on Axis I under DSM-IV guidelines) include Reading Disorder (DSM-IV 315.00), Mathematics Disorder (DSM-IV 315.1) and Disorder Of Written Expression (DSM-IV 315.2).

Mental Retardation and Borderline Intelligence are diagnosed on Axis II in both DSM-III-R and DSM-IV. These are all disorders which place limits on cognitive potential and will produce deficits on neuropsychological examination and limits on the litigant's potential to profit from rehabilitation. Since these disorders are developmental in nature they should not be compensable, but they can be mistakenly attributed to an alleged head injury.

For example, the failure to recognize a plaintiff's pre-existing mental retardation may cause one to over-estimate his or her premorbid functioning, potential to profit from cognitive retraining, and magnify the liability estimate for the insured defendant when in reality the data would not support these conclusions. The identification of these pre-existing conditions is important to the forensic rehabilitation planner.

Axis III

The third axis, Axis III, contains the physical disorders that are relevant to the care, treatment and rehabilitation of the patient. In cases of head injury this may include conditions that are compensable, such as hematomas and seizure disorders. It may also include conditions that affect mentality but which are not compensable, such as degenerative diseases of the central nervous system; vascular disorders; multi-infarct dementia; metabolic, endocrine, and nutritional disorders; endocrinopathies such as hypothyroidism, hypopituitarism, hypoparathyroidism; infections such as meningitis or encephalitis; intoxication from alcohol; and exposure to heavy metals like mercury, lead, arsenic, or thallium. While the cognitive deficits from these factors may be germane to rehabilitation, they would not be a consequence of a head injury and the insurer would have questionable liability for their treatment.

Conditions secondary to the cause of action would be identified here as well. They would clearly have liability for the defendant and would need to be properly identified and addressed. While pre-existing disorders will need to be addressed in treatment their cost would not typically be the responsibility of a third party or defendant.

The identification of all medications taken for conditions listed on this axis and on Axis I would need to be done in the forensic rehabilitation plan. The reason for this is that all medications produce side effects that may be claimed as symptoms secondary to the cause of action. This possibility needs to be accounted for in the treatment plan.

Axis IV

Axis IV, using DSM-III, DSM-III-R and DSM-IV is where psychosocial and environmental stressors are identified. These may be a consequence of injury or they may be pre-existing conditions. Only proper evaluation and discovery will reveal this. All major life stressors should be listed and a cumulative rating is given under DSM-III-R guidelines. Under DSM-IV criteria the psychosocial and environmental stressors are simply listed. Most claimants have multiple sources of life stress that should be considered under Axis IV. Examples of stressors that should be identified and listed here include divorce, unemployment, serious physical injury, and even family arguments. As previously noted, these may be a consequence of injury or pre-existing conditions.

These are important issues to identify and address in a comprehensive treatment/rehabilitation plan. In a forensic rehabilitation plan it will be important to identify whether they are pre-existing or not so as to assign liability.

Axis V

The final axis, Axis V, is for the rating of the patient's level of functioning. It is a composite of social, occupational and recreational activities. It is important to note that many plaintiffs' social profiles have always been constricted and limited by their life-long personality characteristics. In DSM-III-R a 90 point rating scale is utilized and in DSM-IV it has been expanded to a 100 point rating scale. This system is called the Global Assessment of Functioning Scale (GAF). It rates the claimant's current GAF and the highest GAF for the past year. The highest GAF for the past year should actually be considered the goal of the rehabilitation plan and it is not necessary to exceed that level of functioning. For example, if someone was premorbidly Mildly Mentally Retarded, then the goal of the rehabilitation plan should not be to place them in Harvard, train them as a Computer Analyst, or improve their reading ability to the 12th grade level.

Discovery

To fully develop a forensic rehabilitation plan the use of the Discovery process is crucial. Litigants are often poor historians for a variety of reasons, but in any case they are unreliable as to prior diagnosis, treatment, or evaluation issues. The forensic professional will seek to confirm or disconfirm the plaintiff and plaintiff expert claims independently. The only way to do this is through your independent review of all available historical records. If the litigant will not sign releases authorizing one to procure the records, then defense counsel needs to subpoena them during the discovery process. A list of recommended documents to request in discovery includes:

All school records
Marital history
Military records
Employment history
Criminal records
Employment applications
Credit check
Driving record
All hospital records
All pharmaceutical records

All medical evaluation records
All medical treatment notes
All psychiatric, psychological, or neuropsychological treatment notes and billing information
All psychiatric, psychological, or neuropsychological evaluation records including handwritten notes and raw test data.
Insurance claim indexing
Independent examination of the plaintiff

Case Examples

The first case is a claimant seeking damages and rehabilitation for an alleged post concussive syndrome. In this case, there was no loss of consciousness and no positive CT scan, MRI, or EEG to suggest physical damage. When presented with a complete clinical picture, while there is a likely need for treatment and rehabilitation, any compensability for the costs is debatable. There are a number of pre-existing disorders, not counting the side effects of prescribed medication, that could account for all of the plaintiff's reported symptoms. The full multiaxial diagnosis utilizing DSM-III-R guidelines for this plaintiff is as follows:

Axis I:
Dysthymia (DSM-III-R 300.40)
Somatoform Pain Disorder (DSM-III-R 307.80)
Noncompliance With Medical Treatment (DSM-III-R V15.81)
Marital Problem (DSM-III-R V61.10)
Parent-Child Problem (DSM-III-R V61.20)
Uncomplicated Bereavement (DSM-III-R)
Axis II:
Dependent Personality Disorder (DSM-III-R 301.60)
Developmental Reading Disorder (DSM-III-R 315.00)
Axis III:
Migraine Headaches
Arthritis
Obesity

Gastritis
Post Hysterectomy
Hypertension
Possible Irritable Bowel Syndrome

Axis IV:

Psychosocial Stressors:
Marital Conflict Including Physical Abuse
Unemployment
Conflict With Extended Family Members
Litigation
Serious Chronic Illness (migraine headaches and/or depression)
Conflict With Child
Death Of Mother
Severity: Extreme (acute and chronic)

Axis V:

Current GAF: 45
Highest GAF past year: 55

The second case example is a claimant alleging a traumatic brain injury. The following is their complete multiaxial diagnosis using the new DSM-IV guidelines. Since there is documented physical damage (i.e., CT scan, MRI, EEG), some liability is assumed. These disorders identified on the multiaxial system are secondary to the cause of action and treatment and rehabilitation costs are likely compensable.

Axis I:

Amnestic Disorder Due To Head Injury, Chronic Type (DSM-IV 294.0)
Mood Disorder Due To Head Injury With Depressive Features (DSM-IV 293.83)
Partner Relational Problem (DSM-IV V61.1)

Axis II:

No Diagnoses On Axis II (DSM-IV V71.09)

Axis III:

Left Tempo-Parietal Hematoma

Seizure Disorder
Diabetes

Axis IV:

Psychosocial Stressors:
Serious Acute Illness
Unemployment
Serious Financial Problems
Marital Discord

Axis V:

Current GAF: 35
Highest GAF past year: 70

The third case example is a claimant alleging total disability as the result of a claimed closed head injury using both DSM-III-R and DSM-IV multiaxial criteria. Note the placement of the learning disability related disorders In DSM-III-R on Axis II and in DSM-IV on Axis I. There were no documented losses of consciousness or physical evidence of injury, such as MRI, CT scan, or abnormal EEG. A complete multiaxial diagnosis indicated all of her symptoms, physical and mental, were attributable to pre-existing disorders. This multiaxial diagnosis does indicate the need for rehabilitation and treatment, but for pre-existing mental retardation and learning disabilities, and not for a post concussion injury. This multiaxial diagnosis, while suggesting malingering, does not include any compensable injuries.

DSM-III-R

Axis I:

Dysthymia (DSM-III-R 300.40)
Factitious Disorder With Psychological Symptoms (DSM-III-R 300.16)
Malingering (DSM-III-R V65.20)
Noncompliance With Medical Treatment (DSM-III-R V15.81)
Marital Problem (DSM-III-R V61.10)
Parent-Child Problem (DSM-III-R V61.20)

Other Specified Family Circumstances (DSM-III-R 61.80)

Axis II:

Dependent Personality Disorder (DSM-III-R 301.60)
Mild Mental Retardation (DSM-III-R 317.00)
Developmental Arithmetic Disorder (DSM-III-R 315.10)
Developmental Expressive Writing Disorder (DSM-III-R 315.80)
Developmental Reading Disorder (DSM-III-R 315.00)

Axis III:

Amenorrhea
Hirsutism
Chronic Pelvic Pain
Dyspareunia
Right Ectopic Pregnancy
Alopecia

Axis IV:

Birth Of A Child-Gain Of Family Member
Separation-Marital Discord
Surgery
Ectopic Pregnancy
Unemployment
Conflict With Extended Family Members
Litigation
Serious Chronic Illness (retardation and/or depression)
Severity: Extreme (acute and enduring)

Axis V:

Current GAF: 55
Highest GAF past year: 55

DSM-IV

Axis I:

Dysthymia (DSM-IV 300.40)
Factitious Disorder with Predominantly Psychological Symptoms (DSM-IV 300.16)
Malingering (DSM-IV V65.2)

Noncompliance With Medical Treatment (DSM-IV V15.81)
Partner Relational Problem (DSM-III-R V61.1)
Parent-Child Relational Problem (DSM-III-R V61.20)
Relational Problem NOS (DSM-IV V62.81)
Mathematics Disorder (DSM-IV 315.1)
Disorder Of Written Expression (DSM-IV 315.2)
Reading Disorder (DSM-IV 315.00)

Axis II:
Dependent Personality Disorder (DSM-IV 301.6)
Mild Mental Retardation (DSM-IV 317)

Axis III:
Amenorrhea
Hirsutism
Chronic Pelvic Pain
Dyspareunia
Right Ectopic Pregnancy
Alopecia

Axis IV:
Birth Of A Child-Gain Of Family Member
Separation-Marital Discord
Surgery
Ectopic Pregnancy
Unemployment
Conflict With Extended Family Members
Litigation
Serious Chronic Illness (retardation and/or depression)

Axis V:
Current GAF: 55
Highest GAF past year: 55

As the reader can see from the previous case examples the use of the multiaxial diagnostic system recommended in DSM-III, DSM-III-R, and DSM-IV provides a clear straight forward method to comprehensively diagnose claimants' pre-existing and post-cause of action injuries and/or disorders. This comprehensive diagnosis then allows the forensic rehabilitation specialist to develop a prescriptive rehabilitation plan that addresses the claimant's needs while differentiating the compensable injury from the pre-existing disorder.

References

American Psychiatric Association (1980). *Diagnostic and Statistical Manual of Mental Disorders*. Third edition (DSM-III). Washington, D.C.

American Psychiatric Association (1987). *Diagnostic and Statistical Manual of Mental Disorders*. Third edition-revised (DSM-III-R). Washington, D.C.

American Psychiatric Association (1994). *Diagnostic and Statistical Manual of Mental Disorders*. Fourth Edition (DSM IV). Washington, D.C.

Price, D.R. Personality disorders and traits. In McDonald, J.J., Schorring, S.P. & Kulick, F.B. (Eds.). (1994). *Mental and Emotional Injuries in Employment Litigation.* Washington, D.C.: Bureau of National Affairs.

Price, D.R., & Price, D.C. Understanding DSM-III-R, the standard classification system for mental health disorders. In the DRI monograph, *Defending Cases Involving Psychological and Head Injuries*. Vol. 1, Number 3, August 1992.

Regier, D.A., Narrow, W.E., Rae, D.S., Manderscheid, R.W., Locke, B.Z., & Goodwin, F.K. The de facto and addictive disorders service system. *Archives of General Psychiatry*, 50, 85-94.

David R. Price, Ph.D.

Located in Greenville, South Carolina, Dr. Price is a forensic consultant specializing in the defense and limitation of damages for insurance companies, self-insured corporations, and defense counsel across the United States. He is the founder, President, and Senior Analyst of the Insurance/Defense Network. He originated the *Defense of Damages Conference and Seminar and The Annual Symposium on Head Injury Claims,* sponsored by the Insurance/ Defense Network. Dr. Price has published research on diagnostic issues in psychiatric populations and has had extensive clinical experience in diagnosing and treating emotional, organic and mental disorders. Dr. Price was also a founder and principal of one of the largest clinical and consulting psychology practices in South Carolina.

Dr. Price received his undergraduate degree in psychology at Clemson University. He received his Masters and Doctoral degrees in clinical psychology from Auburn University, and interned at the University of Pittsburgh/University Drive VMAC Internship Consortium. Dr. Price is a licensed clinical psychologist with extensive neuropsychological experience and training. Dr. Price has been engaged nationally as a consulting expert in cases ranging from toxic exposure to determination of mitigating circumstances in capital cases. He is a frequent invited lecturer for in-house insurance and law firm seminars, government agencies, bar associations, and claims associations.

In his role as President and Senior Analyst of the Insurance/ Defense Network, Dr. Price specializes in defense case analysis of psychological, neuropsychological, and psychiatric claims in cases including toxic exposure, organic brain syndromes, post traumatic stress disorders, anxiety disorders, and on the presence of factitious disorders and malingering.

4

THE VOCATIONAL EXPERT IN FORENSIC REHABILITATION

Kenneth N. Anchor, Ph.D., ABPP

Medicine, vocational rehabilitation, economics, law, psychology and counseling have all left their mark on the forensic sciences. Some degree of training and experience with each of these fields becomes necessary to work effectively in consulting with courts in matters of personal injury, malpractice, wrongful death and worker's compensation. The adversarial nature of the legal system is often unfamiliar terrain to inexperienced "expert witnesses" often more accustomed to dealing with scientific continual and statistical probabilities.

Vocational consultants are perceived differently by various parties in litigation. The plaintiff attorney looks to the vocational specialist to assist in obtaining the highest possible award for his/her client. The defense attorney employs vocational consultants as a form of damage control to achieve cost containment objectives. Plaintiffs expect vocational consultants to affirm the credibility of their position while defendants anticipate that their experts will discredit the plaintiff by raising issues of malingering, secondary gains, symptom magnification or disincentives to return to work.

Vocational testimony is often essential to laying a foundation for other aspects of litigation. Vocational consultants are often called upon to address the issue of whether or not there has been a diminished earning capacity. This question not only applies to those with a record of employment and earnings history but also to housewives and children.

Customarily, the vocational specialist is called upon to make pre injury versus post-injury comparisons. The court is attempting to assess what would be required in order to restore the individual to being whole and the litigation consultant is assisting in that endeavor.

This chapter will present an overview of the role for vocational testimony in litigation along with a case study.

Understanding Vocational Assessment

The vocational evaluation process is aimed at helping to develop a performance based data set comparing preinjury to post injury work and earning capacity. The assumption is that if a deficit exists, it exists in some amount. When an evaluation is scheduled, the patient should be informed that it will require approximately four to five hours, and if glasses are worn, they should be brought. Ordinarily, the evaluation is conducted in a vocational evaluation performance laboratory but, to an increasing extent, evaluations are scheduled in other cities (hotel rooms, patient homes or attorney offices).

There are four primary components to the evaluation. Initially, a diagnostic interview with a mental status exam will be performed. A patient will be provided an opportunity to describe work history, health circumstances, educational training, relevant family history and lifestyle circumstances. The evaluator has an opportunity to directly observe how the patient communicates, deals with the mild stress of the unfamiliar testing setting and perceives his/her own situation. Some patients are more confident historians than others. Attire, personal hygiene and overall self-presentation may speak volumes about the individual.

The testing segment has three elements. There are a group of standardized work sample procedures or job simulations. These work samples directly measure what a person can and cannot do in simulated work duties. Certainly, the typing test is the best known and one of the very oldest work samples. Once an individual has taken a typing test, actual data have been generated to reduce speculation, assumptions or inference making regarding the individual's capacity to operate a typewriter rapidly and accurately. One might best compare this form of assessment to the use of a dipstick in a motor vehicle to directly evaluate the need for an oil change. These tests function as a dipstick to determine what (marketable) job skills an individual has within his/her repertoire of job skills. Some of these measures are administered sitting, while others are administered standing up. Some involve writing while others do not.

A second group of tests deals with mental ability. Intelligence test batteries assist in evaluating a level of intellectual functioning (and percentile or range), judgment, reasoning, concentration, and memory or related cognitive abilities. Since intelligence is one of the two most important factors generally examined by prospective employers, this is a key part of the testing process. Many of these measures are timed.

The final stage of the evaluation includes personality testing. Several psychological measures are included to determine whether or not the individual meets the criteria for a diagnosable mental disorder. If psychopathology or serious maladjustment can be ruled out, this should be a favorable predictor for entry or re-entry into the market.

The research literature indicates that a small percentage of individuals do attempt to be manipulative, deceptive or dishonest. It is a frequently asked question of vocational evaluators, "how do you know the person has given good effort on these tests?" Fortunately, the field of psychometric testing has addressed this critical issue in several ways. There are symptom magnification instruments which lend themselves to inclusion in such an assessment. The best known and most widely used personality measure, the Minnesota Multiphasic Personality Inventory, has a Lie Scale built into its format which includes ten clinical scales in addition to three validity scales that aim at helping to detect the malingerer or person whose behavior is being shaped by secondary gains. Other tests focus upon credibility (i.e., creating the opportunity to respond inconsistently).

Though it is true that in recent years the Supreme Court has disallowed polygraph testing for most types of employment screening, most psychological testing has withstood the scrutiny of government watchdog agencies. One of the most difficult aspects of dealing with this arena is that while some individuals may be intentionally exaggerating or overreacting to symptoms, others do so unintentionally. Of course, one of the greatest assets of having experienced clinicians perform such a battery of tests is that they can buttress test findings by using their own clinical judgment in exposing dishonest or fraudulent patients. Ordinarily, this author uses two or three such credibility measures as a part of a comprehensive test battery.

Foundations for Vocational Perspective

The experienced vocational specialist frequently provides a wealth of information regarding opportunities for vocational rehabilitation, work hardening/enhancement, pain management, cognitive retraining, recreational therapy, transportation services for the disabled, practical home modifications, occupational therapy, job placement and other avenues for helping to successfully rehabilitate injured parties, and the costs associated with those services and equipment. The recent passage of the Americans with Disabilities Act (ADA) may go a long way toward enlarging opportunities for individuals with various deficits to successfully re-enter society with little or no stigma in the future. This legislation is aimed at ringing the death knell on both overt and covert employer biases toward previously injured job applicants.

The economics of rehabilitation analysis should be carefully considered. Preventive measures almost certainly yield substantial savings. Taking rapid and responsible action with a long-term strategy often proves invaluable. Understanding the marked difference between medical impairments and vocational disability rating has far-reaching implications. It must be recognized that misleading statistics and spurious assumptions produce incorrect conclusions. A subtle but sometimes critical dimension of litigation analysis of personal injury, malpractice, and workers' compensation is the impact of prior injuries or pre-existing health problems. The vocational specialist has an array of tools to help systematically assign meaningful values to the appropriate cause when requested to do so.

An understanding of the labor market is essential to functioning effectively as a vocational consultant. Hiring standards and practices vary across industries and may be directly affected by cycles of the economy. A challenge frequently confronted by vocational specialists in litigation is how best to communicate technical information. In this regard, the federal government did the public a great service when it sponsored the Department of Labor to establish a *Dictionary of Occupational Titles* to classify all jobs in the U.S. economy according to several salient dimensions. Jurors and others will readily grasp that all jobs fall into one of five categories ranging from sedentary to very heavy types of exertion.

Category of Work Exertion	Percentage of Jobs
Sedentary	10.96%
Light	49.59%
Medium	29.59%
Heavy	9.14%
Very Heavy	.72%

VOCATIONAL READINGS

Another critical part of the vocational consultant's conceptual framework is to understand the role of specific vocational preparation required for any given job. The amount of time needed to learn the work duties, acquire the pertinent information and develop the facility for average performance in a specific job-worker situation that meets minimal employer requirements for productivity are all important considerations. Specific vocational preparation may derive from formal educational training background, military and institutional work experience, apprenticeship or on-the-job training. Based upon the system established by the U.S. Department of Labor, there are nine levels used for determining how best to rate each job. Those levels are as follows with the actual proportion of jobs requiring such a background shown in parenthesis:

Unskilled one (1.5%) short demonstration only
Unskilled two (23.03%) up to 30 days
Semi-skilled three (17.26%) 30 days to 3 months
Semi-skilled four (12.85%) 3 to 6 months
Skilled five (9.46%) 6 months to 1 year
Skilled six (10.42%) 1 to 2 years (Certification/AA)
Skilled seven (16.13%) 2 to 4 years (AA/BA/BS)
Highly skilled eight (8.99%) 4 to 10 years (MS/Ph.D.)
Highly skilled nine (.36%) over 10 years

In determining what jobs a disabled individual is capable of performing, one's aptitudes must be considered with eleven of the most important aptitudes predictive of employability as follows:

General Learning Ability - General ability to learn, reason and make judgments
Verbal - Ability to understand and use words effectively
Numerical - Ability to understand and perform mathematical functions
Spatial - Ability to visualize three dimension objects from two
Form Perception - Ability to perceive and distinguish graphic detail
Clerical Perception - Ability to see and distinguish verbal detail
Motor Coordination - Ability to coordinate eyes, hands and fingers
Finger Dexterity - Ability to finger and manipulate small objects
Manual Dexterity - Ability to handle, place and turn motions

Eye/Hand/Foot Coordination - Motor responsiveness to visual stimuli
Color Discrimination - Ability to match/discriminate colors

There are a great many tests available for evaluating individuals alleging a disability which interferes with their work capacity. Among the most frequently used tests are the following:

Adult Basic Learning Examination (ABLE)
American College Testing Program Exam
Attitude and Competency Sections
Basic Skills Test
Beck Depression Inventory
Bennett Hand Tool Work Sample
Benton Visual Retention Test, Revised Edition
Business Education Achievement Tests
California Achievement Tests
California Life Goals Evaluation Schedule
California Occupational Preference
California Psychological Inventory (CPI)
Career Assessment Inventory
Career Directions Inventory
Comrey Personality Inventory
Computer Aptitude, Literacy and Interest Profile
Crawford Small Parts Dexterity Test
Culture Fair Intelligence Test
Diagnostic Reading Tests
Daily Stress Inventory
Differential Aptitude Tests
Differential Aptitude Tests Fifth Edition
Dr. Paul Lees-Haley Credibility Scale
Edwards Personal Preference Schedule (EPPS)
Embedded Figures Test
Employee Aptitude Survey
Error Proneness Scale
Flanagan Aptitude Classification Tests (FACT)
Flanagan Industrial Tests
Forer Vocational Survey: Men-Women
Fundamental Interpersonal Relations Orientation Behavior (FIRO-B)
General Aptitude Test Battery (GATB)
Geist Picture Interest Inventory

Goldstein-Scheerer Tests of Abstract and Concrete Thinking
Gordon Occupational Check List II
Gordon Personal Inventory
Guildford-Zimmerman Aptitude Test
Guildford-Zimmerman Interest Inventory
Guildford-Zimmerman Temperament Survey
Hall Occupational Orientation Inventory
Halstead-Reitan Neuropsychological Screening Battery
Hand-Tool Dexterity Test
Haptic Intelligence Scale
Hogan Personality Inventory
Holland Vocational Preference Inventory
Holmes and Rabe Social Readjustment Scale
Human Activity Profile
Illinois Test of Psycholinguistic Ability
The Interest Check List
Iowa Tests of Basic Skills
Iowa Tests of Educational Development
Jackson Vocational Interest Survey
Jenkins Activity Scale
Kahn Intelligence Test
Kohn Block Design Test
Kuder General Interest Survey
Kuder Occupational Interest Survey
Leisure Activities Blank
Leiter International Performance Scale
Luria-Nebraska Neuropsychological Battery
MacGuarrie Test for Mechanical Ability Seashore-Bennett Stenographic Proficiency Test
Marlow-Crowne Need for Social Approval Scale
Maslach Burnout Inventory
McGill Pain Questionnaire
Test of Mechanical Ability
Memory-for-Designs Test
(Graham-Kendall)
Metropolitan Achievement Test
Millon Behavioral Health Inventory
Millon Clinical Multiaxial Inventory
Millon Clinical Multiaxial Inventory - II
Minnesota Clerical Tests
Minnesota Counseling Inventory
Minnesota Multiphasic Personality Inventory
Minnesota Multiphasic Personality Inventory 2

Revised Minnesota Paper Form Board Test
Minnesota Rate of Manipulation Tests
Minnesota Spatial Relations Test Revised Edition
Minnesota Vocational Interest Inventory
Modern Language Aptitude Test
Motor-Free Visual Perception Test
Multiaxial Diagnostic Inventory
Multidimensional Aptitude Battery
Multiple Affect Adjective Checklist
Musical Aptitude Survey and Interest Schedule (OASIS)
Occupational Literacy
Occupational Stress Inventory
Ohio Vocational Interest Survey-Second Edition
Otis Employment Test
Otis-Lennon Mental Ability Test
Peabody Picture Vocabulary Test - Revised
Peabody Individual Achievement Test - Revised
Pennsylvania Bi-Manual Work Sample
Performax Scales
Personal Orientation Inventory
Personality Research Form
Portable Assessment Systems
Productivity Environmental Preference Survey
Psycho-Social Pain Inventory
Purdue Creativity Test
Purdue Pegboard
Purdue Personnel Tests
Quick Neuropsychological Screening Test
Quick Test
Raven Progressive Matrices
Reading-Free Vocational Interest Inventory
Rey Auditory-Verbal Learning Test
Rosenzweig Picture Frustration Study
Rotter Incomplete Sentences Blank
Rush Cognitive Screening Battery
Seashore Measures of Musical Talents, Revised Edition
Self-Directed Search
Senior Apperception Test
Shipley Institute of Living Scale - Revised
Short Employment Tests
Short Tests of Clerical Ability
Sixteen Personality Factor Questionnaire
Slosson Intelligence Test

Speilberger State/Trait Anxiety Inventory
SRA Typing Skills
Standardized Work Performance Sample Procedures
Stanford-Binet Intelligence Test - Revised
Stromberg Dexterity Test
Strong-Campbell Interest Inventory
Study of Values
Survey of Work Styles
Systematic Approach to Vocational Evaluation (S.A.V.E.)
Tactual Performance Test
Tactual Progressive Matrices
Temperament and Values Inventory
Test of Non-Verbal Intelligence
Test of Non-Verbal Intelligence - 2
Test in Fundamental Abilities Visual Arts
Revised Token Test
Torrance Tests of Creative Thinking
Turse Clerical Aptitudes Test
USES Interest Inventory
Valpar Component Work Samples 1-16
Vineland Adaptive Behavior Scales
Vineland Social Maturity Scale
Visual Form Discrimination
Vocational Adaptation Rating Scales
Vocational Preference Inventory
Wahler Physical Symptoms Inventory
Watson-Glaser Critical Thinking Appraisal
Wechsler Adult Intelligence Scale - Revised (WAIS-R)
Wechsler Memory Scale - Revised
Wesman Personnel Classification Test
WEST #1
WEST #2
WEST #3
WEST #4
WEST #5
Wide Range Achievement Tests - Revised
Wide Range Intelligence and Personality Test
Wide Range Interest and Opinion Tests
Wonderlic Personnel Test
Zung Depression Scale

Case Study

The following case study incorporates each of these elements discussed in this chapter and are all intended to provide an overview of the areas in which a vocational consultant might be called upon to testify. The first report is based upon about a half day evaluation which includes testing and a diagnostic interview. This evaluation yields a disability rating, if any is warranted. The second report presents a diminished earning capability study which outlines the amount of loss the injured party can be expected to lose.

Vocational and Psychological Evaluation

Patient: John Doe
Date Of Birth: September 10, 1950
Date Administered: January 15, 1993
Test Administered: Standardized Work Performance Sample Procedures; Shipley-Hartford Institute of Living Scale-Revised Norms; WEST Tool Sort; Flanagan Industrial Test; Performance Assessment and Capacity Test; Multiaxial Diagnostic Inventory; Minnesota Multiphasic Personality Inventory-2; Stress Audit; Error Proneness; Wahler Physical Symptoms Inventory; Physical Complaints Survey Schedule (partial); Loma Linda University Activity Scale; Credibility Scale; Push/Pull Exertional Scale; Incomplete Sentences Blank and Diagnostic Interview.
Documents Reviewed: Medical Records; Hospital Records

Background And Behavioral Observations:

Mr. Doe was born and currently resides in ________________ county. His father worked as a desalinization technician and his mother as a factory worker. He is the oldest of five children. This individual is right handed. His formal educational training includes a high school diploma (honor roll) and two years of college studies at Community College where he reportedly majored in Marine Construction and earned an associate's degree with a grade point average of about 3.4. He also earned a real estate license after having taken several courses in that field of study about 10 years ago.

For the past 20 years, he has been married to a computer operator but has been separated for about one year. He is the father of three children (ages 7, 14 and 19).

Mr. Doe was somewhat evasive during the lengthy assessment process. He seemed inclined to give partial answers to questions which had to be repeated for him. He rarely made eye contact. Initially, he seemed to complain at every opportunity. It was observed that he sat for nearly two hours being interviewed and completing various tests before the examiner suggested a break. Mr. Doe encountered no difficulties in comprehending test instructions. Some of the information he provided was inconsistent. He seemed quite blameful toward others. Toward the latter stages of the evaluation, a greater degree of rapport was established.

Mr. Doe has been gainfully employed in different capacities during his career including having held jobs as electrician's helper, jewelry store clerk, field engineer and letter carrier for the Postal Service for approximately 16 years. According to the U.S. Department of Labor's *Dictionary of Occupational Titles* and the *Encyclopedia of Job Requirements*, most of Mr. Doe's prior relevant work assignments have required light or medium work exertion. He recalled having served two years in the U.S. Army as an ammunition technician. He denied ever being fired or terminated from a position. Based on figures presented in the *American Almanac of Jobs and Salaries*, Mr. Doe has generally earned in the average range of compensation for most of his prior jobs. During 1987 and 1988, he served as a relief supervisor, responsible for approximately 30 employees. More recently, Mr. Doe has received training to audit books for the postal service and in the past had also received training as an accident investigator for the postal service.

Mr. Doe described his health circumstances. While serving in the Army in Vietnam, he suffered from hypertension and contracted hepatitis. He has used marijuana and has a history of drinking (primarily beer). In approximately 1982, he was treated for back pain. As a child, he had a collapsed lung. He was treated in approximately 1969 for problems with his right foot. As early as 1972, he complained of back pain. In 1973, he learned that he had sickle cell trait. In 1973, his veteran's records indicate problems with interpersonal relationships and chronic severe anxiety which manifested themselves in psychosomatic complaints. He was diagnosed with a nervous disorder, shoulder condition and anemia. In 1976, he complained of heart problems. Bouts of severe anger were detected along with anxiety episodes in 1976 and psychiatric treatment as recommended at that time. In 1980, he presented with varicose veins. Back spasms occurred in 1982 which required treatment. In 1982, while boating, he injured his back. Subsequently, he broke his wrist while at work delivering the mail. Records indicate treatment for phlebitis. Mr. Doe reported that several spinal headaches developed following a mylogram. In 1983, he was readmitted for back pain problems. In 1984, Mr. Doe was in a motor vehicle accident. No surgery was required. He did receive physical therapy and medications. He remained off work for two to three weeks before returning to limited duty and continued to work on a part-time basis for about one year. He reported suffering a seizure and did not work at all for about two years. Presently, he works four hours a day as a postal clerk and has done so since February, 1992. He denied any falling or problems with his balance. He denied suicidal ideation. Mr. Doe indicated that he has been seizure free since March, 1992. Mr. Doe's father was an alcoholic and he also began drinking at an early age and was arrested for drinking at the age of 16. He reported that he continues to drink but would not be specific as to how much and how often.

Mr. Doe described his range of activities and lifestyle. Ordinarily, he might rise about 5:30 a.m., drive himself to work, eat at the post office, work from 6:30 to 10:30 a.m., go home, fix a meal, do light housekeeping, take out the garbage, wash the dishes, take his laundry to his mother, sweep, make the bed, use the telephone, shop, put gas in the car, watch TV, rest, go for a walk and go to bed. He is able to manage his own money and look after his personal needs. For leisure, he enjoys walking, swimming, travel, movies, attending yard sales and watching his 14 year old play Little League baseball. He also attends church. Since he is estranged from his wife, Mr. Doe lives alone. On weekends, he said he prefers to "lay around the house." Other activities which Mr. Doe indicated he is satisfactorily able to perform include using various items and tools such as grocery basket, spatula, mop, dust cloth, utensils, blow dryer, shaving items, pots, trays, skillet, hoe, knife, rake, stapler, sponge, scraper, hole punch, spray can, pitcher, pen, slotted screw driver, shears, wrench, scrub brush, electric drill, paint brush, shovel, hand drill, locking pliers, hog ringer pliers, lineman's pliers, ratchet screw driver, pincer pliers, electrical pliers, cable cutter, torque wrench, all purpose pliers, longnose pliers, crescent adjustable wrench, diagonal cutting pliers, C-clamp, wire stripping pliers, crimping pliers, open end wrench, nut driver screw driver, hammer, household broom and push broom.

In looking to the future, Mr. Doe stated he would like to return to full-time work and "get on with my life." He has inquired into other jobs and is currently considering returning to real estate: "everyone said I was so good at it." He also expressed an interest in working at a travel related job.

Test Results:

The following testing methods were conducted with Mr. Doe in accordance with the standards and procedures recommended by the American Board of Professional Disability Consultants. The composite test findings obtained from the administration of the Standardized Work Performance Sample Procedures revealed the following:

Work Tolerance Under Loan:	Average
Foot Pedal Operation:	Average
Grip Strength:	Average
Arm/Hand Steadiness:	Above Average
Assembly/Disassembly (Timed standing and seated):	Average

Manual Dexterity:	Average
Error Proneness:	Average
Job Material Sorting (Timed standing and seated):	Average
Ability to Deal with Stressful Work Circumstances:	Average
Transferability of Skills (based on present residual functional capacity):	Above Average
Freedom from Distractibility:	Average

(The rating categories are as follows):

Very Superior:	(96-99th Percentile)
Superior:	(84-95th Percentile)
Above Average:	(62-83rd Percentile)
Average:	(39-61st Percentile)
Below Average:	(17-38th Percentile)
Poor:	(5-16th Percentile)
Very Poor:	(1-4th Percentile)

Mr. Doe achieved an I.Q. test score which places him in the average range of intellectual functioning. His ability to sustain attention and concentration was not impaired. Problem solving skills are stable. No limitations were detected for logic, judgment and reasoning. His ability to sustain attention and concentration is within average limits. Mental alertness is in the average range. No clinically remarkable cognitive deficits were identified.

Mr. Doe's test responses are not indicative of a diagnosable mental disorder or psychopathology. He appears to be satisfactorily adjusting to his current circumstances. He demonstrates a capacity to establish and maintain relationships. Some patients with similar test profiles have a tendency to be preoccupied with symptomatology and may overreact to it. He appears to understand his own limitations but demonstrated a limited degree of self-insight. Reality contact is good. Psychological defenses are adequate to cope with the demands and stressors of daily living but he may occasionally engage in self-defeating behavior. Symptom magnification, malingering and secondary gains could not be ruled out by these test data.

Conclusions and Recommendations:

Test findings are felt to be valid and reliable.

Mr. Doe does not meet the criteria for a diagnosable mental disorder and did not exhibit clinical signs or symptoms reflective of serious psychological maladjustment. He is effectively adapting to and compensating for his current circumstances. Credibility findings for this individual are questionable as it appears he may have been seeking to intentionally or unintentionally be manipulative to certain test responses. Presently, Mr. Doe demonstrates mild vocational limitations and should be considered to have an industrial/occupational disability rating of 12-17% (that is, of the pool of jobs which he could have satisfactorily performed prior to his recent health circumstances, he retains the ability to perform 83-88% of that pool of jobs if sufficiently motivated to return to full-time gainful employment). He appears to possess the vocational capacity and transferable skills to perform a full range of sedentary and light work assignments which would be within his range of capabilities. It appears that Mr. Doe does not seem to be motivated or interested in returning to full-time gainful employment at this time. Individuals with this test profile are often ambivalent about returning to work. This younger worker possesses transferable job skills which would be readily marketable if he chose to seriously pursue a return to work. It is recommended that he receive short-term counseling (available through his employee assistance program) to enable him to work through some of his personal concerns and outpatient pain management rehabilitation services to assist him in more effectively coping with his physical complaints.

Projected Future Earnings: Loss Report

Patient: John Doe
Date Of Birth: September 10, 1950
Date Of Report: January 20, 1993
Resource Materials:

Various Publications of Upjohn Institute for Employment Research
American Almanac of Jobs and Salaries
Work Life Expectancy Table
Handbook for Analyzing Jobs
National Employment Projections
The Vocational Expert
Classification of Jobs
A Guide to Job Analysis
Labor Market Access
Probability of Labor Force participation
Economic Insights
Determining Disability and Worth
Handbook of Labor Statistics
Tables of Working Life
New Work Life Estimates
Employment and Earnings
U.S. Chamber of Commerce Employee Benefits
Consumer Expenditure Survey Series
National Data Book and Guide to Resources
Vocational and Psychological
Evaluation: January 15, 1993

To perform such an analysis one must consider Mr. Doe's residual vocational capacity for successful gainful employment and work adjustment. The establishment of the residual earning capacity must address the manner in which the functional limitations may be imposed by an injury. A pre-injury and post-injury capacity comparison is made relative to earning capacity.

A determination of the economic value of career earnings is involved in some cases of physical impairment. The evaluation process involves: a) estimating what the income stream would have been for Mr. Doe without the vocational limitations, b) estimating the residual earning capacity, or what Mr. Doe will be able to do now.

Initial determination may be based upon Mr. Doe's residual capacity, that is, a profile of his physical abilities considering the existing limitation(s) and the profile matched against job requirements. If the pre-existing limitations are intellectual, an estimate can be made of the probable effect upon academic achievement and the capacity established based on this determination. The establishment of the residual earning capacity involves finding answers to the questions of:

1. What jobs a person is or will be capable of doing?
2. How likely is it that the individual can find employment in those jobs?
3. What is the pay scale for the types of jobs the person is capable of doing?

The functional limitations imposed by the injury considered are the major determinants of the opportunities available to Mr. Doe for vocational alternatives. Minimal employment would assume the current federal minimum wage level of $4.25 per hour. The difference between pre-injury and post-injury work and earning capacity are central considerations for such a projection in regard to Mr. Doe.

The extent of the vocational economic effects may be estimated by establishing a profile of Mr. Doe <u>without</u> the physical and/or mental limitation and a profile <u>with</u> the limitation. The profiles can then be matched against worker requirements for jobs in the national economy to determine what proportion of the jobs Mr. Doe could have performed but cannot now perform with the limitation in such a way that would meet minimal employer expectations. The percentage of the jobs from which the individual has been eliminated may be used as an estimate of the occupational disability. The recent enactment of the Americans with Disabilities Act must be considered along with its far reaching implications for the disabled job candidate.

Taking into account all favorable and unfavorable factors, it appears that Mr. Doe may experience modest career earnings capacity loss. His pre-injury earnings capacity to age 65 would have been $1,105,770. This figure assumes a supplement to earnings/fringe benefit level of 23%. His pre-injury earning capacity to age 62 would have been $998,760 using the same 23% rate of fringe benefits.

Current post-injury status for Mr. Doe indicates that he presently retains the capacity to earn 3% ($33,173) to 8% ($88,462) less than he would have earned with no injury resulting from the motor vehicle accident to age 65. Using a career life expectancy projection to age 62 the figures would be as follows: 3% ($29,963) to 8% ($79,901) less than he would have earned without the injury. In view of his lengthy medical history which predates the work related injury, some portion of these projected losses may be attributable to premorbid factors and to post accident problems which do not appear to be a result of the motor vehicle accident.

These projections have been discounted to present value using the total offset approach based upon equivalence between inflation and average annual pay increases.

Professional Qualifications

For vocational consultants who engage in forensic work, credentialing and certification is growing in importance. Since expertise as a vocational specialist is interdisciplinary in nature involving a working knowledge of psychology, rehabilitation, economics, medicine and even some law, no single discipline can claim ownership. There are organizations which have been established to monitor standards for practice, ethical guidelines, certification procedures and continuing education program requirements. The American Board of Professional Disability

Consultants is one such organization with which many vocational specialists are affiliated and have been recognized for board certification.

Many vocational consultants work closely with various government agencies. Some consultants review files to help determine whether or not a claimant meets the criteria for an entitlement program. Others are called upon to appear at administrative hearings to answer hypothetical questions and provide information with regard to a claimant's past work history and transferable job skills (if any). Such individuals are often under contract and rotated randomly for various hearings. Many individuals who do this as a major thrust of their career have primary training backgrounds in rehabilitation or psychology. Vocational specialists have a close working familiarity with the governmental regulations pertinent to making decisions regarding individual applicants for programs funded by State and Federal agencies. In addition to exertional impairment, nonexertional impairments are frequently involved. Nonexertional impairments do not limit physical exertion and do not directly affect one's ability to sit, stand, walk, lift, push, carry or pull. These include disorders affecting the mind, vision, hearing, speech and use of the body to balance, stoop, climb, kneel, crawl, crouch, handle, reach and have dexterous and bilateral use of the hands and fingers for fine motor manipulation activities.

With increasing frequency, vocational specialists find themselves consulting in cases dealing with personal injury, wrongful death, malpractice, workman's compensation and malpractice. Since plaintiff attorneys must initiate a court action, they are usually the first to search out vocational consultants. However, there has been a growing trend by defense attorneys to readily counter with a vocational consultant of their own. Too often, they have found themselves at a disadvantage if the plaintiff has engaged the services of a vocational specialist and their side has not done so.

Vocational Consultants in Litigation

Qualified vocational specialists are broadly trained and function in a variety of forensic and consultative roles. Recent trends in some regions indicate that a defense posture gaining acceptance is to "fight fire with fire." That is, rather than overlooking that the plaintiff is relying upon vocational testimony, the defendants are beginning to seek out their own vocational evidence. Vocational specialists can assist litigation in various ways, among which are the following:

1. Establish the presence or absence of a disability (and its extent) based upon the use of statistically valid and scientifically reliable assessment procedures.
2. Explain and articulate the economic consequences of a disability (if any).
3. Help to provide authorization rehabilitation analysis regarding the worth of the case and the settlement value of a matter in litigation (e.g., the worth of a life in a wrongful death matter).
4. Assist in identifying preventive and proactive steps to settle litigation in a constructive, reasonable and timely fashion.
5. Serve as a liaison between the allegedly injured or disabled individual and (prospective) employers (for example, oftentimes, employers are willing to take an injured worker back but require assistance and assurance that job modification will successfully minimize safety or other risk factors for the employee).
6. Help to identify malingerers, symptom magnifiers, manipulators and others motivated either intentionally or unintentionally by secondary gains and/or financial incentives.
7. Help to organize a comprehensive rehabilitation treatment plan, as well as possible sources to provide those services along with a range of costs (for example, a Life Care Plan).

8. Help to evaluate the significance of the treatment issues (short-term versus long-term; inpatient versus outpatient).
9. Help to diagnose individuals who may be overreacting to situational stress.
10. Help to designate which individuals are ready to return to work (for example, part-time or lighter duties) in a way that could be therapeutic in accelerating recovery.
11. Help to discern what transferable skills an individual may possess and how they may be useful in returning that individual to the labor market for substantial gainful employment.

Understanding Vocational Economics

Vocational economics is a frequently misunderstood aspect of examining damages. If there are real damages, there are ways of measuring or ascertaining what those damages are in financial terms. There are several economic models for analyzing loss of wages and benefits in cases of injury. The purpose of this chapter is not to focus upon that subject but some of the more frequently encountered models are the total offset approach, present value approach and the inflation discount/real interest method. In some instances, a particular model, such as the total offset method, may be mandated in a particular jurisdiction. Different vocational economists will argue for the merits of one model over another. However, the thrust of any paradigm concerning damages is to determine a realistic and sensible way to restore the injured party to being whole once again. Awards made for damages, pain and suffering and loss of consortium are above and beyond the issue of actual loss.

Any vocational economist will be quick to point out that in order to best understand economic matters, one must look at a long period of time, such as several decades in order to detect meaningful trends. An aberration of the economy in a one or two year period should not overshadow the ebb and flow of long-term economic cycles.

The average person will easily comprehend that a dollar in 1950 bought far more than a dollar buys today. The same logic dictates that today's dollar is more powerful than will be the value of the dollar in 25 years. Consequently, careful economic projections need to take into account interest rates and how they affect purchasing power. Fortunately, various governmental agencies using large statistical basis make available data which aid in such calculations.

Another factor of considerable importance is fringe benefits or supplements to earnings. According to the U.S. Chamber of Commerce there has been an upward trend (which may be peaking now) for fringe benefits. Fringe benefits may be defined in different ways but according to that same organization the average American worker received in excess of 30 percent in fringe benefits. Since fringe benefits do not show up on the paycheck, they should not be overlooked. On the other hand, it is important that those figures not be inflated unreasonably.

Vocational experts often provide input with regard to the extent of financial damage which may have been suffered by an individual. Age, education, work history, lifestyle and health circumstances (both before and after the accident of health setback) are considered. One of the few surveys of settlement awards was published in a law journal a decade ago and revealed that the average amount of financial settlement per case was $64,116. The range of awards according to the type of injury is shown in Table 4.1.

Some ingenuity and creativity is necessary. It is important to determine what local resources may be available to help become familiar with local hiring standards and practices. Vocational consultants are expected to know rates of unemployment as well as major employers in any given area. Libraries, medical center and Chamber of Commerce offices often have useful data available. State and Federal agencies (for example, Bureau of Labor Statistics, Department of Census and State Departments of Labor) often publish surveys of considerable interest.

It is recommended that vocational consultants become familiar with local economists and collect data dealing with

TABLE 4.1 *Settlement Awards*

Area Injury	# Cases	Range	Mean
Brain	29	$750 - 2,744,059	$283,063
Face & Skull	68	50 - 2,275,000	50,966
Shoulder	20	250 - 300,953	38,190
Arm & Elbow	36	50 - 425,000	44,458
Wrist & Hand	29	2000 - 281,000	36,851
Neck & Cervical	120	350 - 649,481	30,846
General Back	90	500 - 830,000	44,452
Lumbar & Low Back	63	500 - 412,000	74,000
Internal Injuries	22	314 - 800,000	99,631
Hip & Pelvis	10	500 - 200,000	61,120
Leg & Foot	69	1000 - 325,000	72,828
Knee	22	200 - 250,000	49,686
Loss of Senses	10	10,000 - 500,000	89,250
Sexual Injuries	5	1250 - 250,000	56,950
Burns	18	4000 - 1,000,000	326,286
Other	64	300 - 638,000	30,049

Average settlement per case = $64,116
Source: *Loyola Law Review* (1982,1983)
Cases 1979-1983

vocational economics. It is useful to purchase books (for example, *American Almanac of Jobs and Salaries*) and subscribe to relevant journals (for example, *Journal of Forensic Economics*), as well as attend conferences, seminars and workshops dealing with diminished earnings issues. Auditing courses in labor economics at local universities and related subjects can be quite helpful. Of course, collaborating with local economists can be enormously instructive. The language of vocational economics is somewhat different than most helping professionals are familiar with, and one is encouraged to read actual reports.

Some of the U.S. Department of Labor's publications that are frequently used as resources are the following:

1. *The Dictionary of Occupational Titles*
2. *A Guide to Job Analysis*

3. *Guide to Occupational Exploration*
4. *Monthly Labor Review*
5. *Occupational Outlook Handbook*
6. Selected characteristics of occupations defined in *The Dictionary of Occupational Titles*

Some of the more helpful publications generated by the Bureau of Labor Statistics are:

1. *Area Wage Surveys* (for standard Metropolitan statistical areas)
2. *Consumer Price Index Detailed Report* (monthly)
3. *Employment and Earnings* (monthly)
4. *Current Wage Developments* (monthly data on consumer price index)
5. *Employment and Earnings Supplement*
6. *Employment Hours and Earnings, States and Areas*
7. *Employment Hours and Earnings, United States*
8. *Industry Wage Surveys* (for selected industries)
9. *List of Unskilled, Light and Sedentary Occupations*

Emerging Role of Vocational Consultant - TBI

Vocational specialists frequently engage in training, research and consultation dealing with traumatic brain injury. The young field of neuropsychology, the study of brain/behavior relationships, is rapidly defining itself with voluminous research. Factors in neuropsychological evaluation frequently include assessment of the following:

1. Attention/Concentration/Freedom from distractibility
2. Capacity of information processing
3. Speed of information processing
4. Short and long-term memory
5. Capacity for learning new skills
6. Abstract thinking

7. Problem solving
8. Communication skills
9. Visuospatial skills
10. Perceptual skills
11. Executive functions
12. Emotional functioning
13. Social functioning
14. Personality functioning

A conventional profile may encompass only four general categories for rating each of these neuropsychological factors: No Deficits, Mild Deficits, Moderate Deficits or Severe Deficits. However, a comprehensive rehabilitation analysis would also include another critically important category for study: Pseudo-deficits. Methods of detecting individuals who seek to deceive, distort or otherwise misrepresent themselves have gained a stronghold in the behavior sciences that measures up well under scientific scrutiny (unlike polygraph testing which has been largely disallowed by the U.S. Supreme Court for purposes of determining suitability for employment).

Disability management is a dynamic, proactive process of minimizing the impact of injury, disability or disease on a worker's capacity to perform work effectively, safely and reliably. It requires the active planning and coordination of labor, management, insurance carriers, health care providers and vocational consultants. It is a strategy for orchestrating and closely monitoring all aspects of returning an injured person to the work force, including tracking medical treatment, motivation for work return and identifying and resulting barriers to work return. Disability management promotes disability prevention, strategies, rehabilitation treatment concepts and safe work return programs designed to control the personal and economic costs of work place injury.

Soft tissue injuries are the most common and costly year after year. The National Safety Council reports that about 2% of the entire work force suffers from a back injury each year. However, this is not a homogeneous group since some individuals continue working, some seek rehabilitation treatment and others become litigious. Before World War II, spinal cord injury was usually a lethal condition. Recently, methods of management of every affected body system have dramatically improved, significantly reducing mortality and allowing for a prospect of a greatly enhanced quality of life for the spinal cord injury patient. With open or closed head injuries, it is critical to be able to describe the prognosis and implications for everyday functioning in very practical terms. The eighteen-month follow-up assessment is important because most recovery will have occurred by that time; further recovery will probably be minimal and extended over a much longer period. The foundation for addressing such issues is no longer narrowly medical. Rather, it is seen as a broader vocational and neuropsychologic concern most effectively addressed by vocational specialists with recognized expertise in job placement, rehabilitation, psychodiagnostics, vocational forecasting and work tolerance, possessing a current fund of knowledge in neurobehavioral science research.

The vast majority of patients with mild head trauma are between the ages of 16 and 29. Children can experience head trauma with very different consequences from those of their adult counterparts. Intelligence generally does not stabilize until about the age of twelve for most persons and the younger that injured child, the less certain one can be in predicting potential or capacity for adult cognitive functioning. In such instances, projections become largely based on parents' work and earnings history, education, economic indications, work life expectancy and related data.

Delayed Recovery/Magnification of Illness Behavior

There are various non-medical explanations to explain a delayed recovery:

1. Psychological stressors (fear of re-injury, marital problems or child related concerns at home)
2. Socially unacceptable disabilities which are masked or

concealed (substance abuse crisis underlying a low back pain ruse)
3. Career dissatisfaction or burnout (underlying objective to locate a different job)
4. Employer and labor relations issues (desire to penalize the supervisor)
5. Legal issues (desire for financial settlement)

Further, potential causes for magnified illness behavior include:

1. Unrecognized severity of the patient's pathologic condition
2. Psychologic distress related to the duration, nature and/or failure of treatment
3. Intense job dissatisfaction
4. Dislike of the supervisor or employer
5. Voluntary exaggeration to influence mediolegal proceedings

Clinical experience is instructive regarding those who claim to suffer from chronic pain syndrome. Among the pattern of characteristics exhibited by patients with this profile are the following:

1. Inconsistency of pain presentation from one evaluation session to the next
2. Pain tends to be global affecting multiple, unrelated areas which do not correspond to any anatomic or physiologic pathology
3. Alleged discomfort is not related to a discrete area but rather total body discomfort
4. Diminished level of overall activity or selective inactivity
5. Unproductive, overutilization of health care need rehabilitation resources
6. History of psychological maladjustment
7. Litigation in process
8. Secondary gain or other disincentives to resume employment.

The absence of early and ongoing communication between the employer and the disabled employee is a serious omission on the part of employers which may impede an employee's return to work. A great many workers alleging injury feel personally let down when employers and supervisors fail to express concern, support or otherwise show reasonable interest in the person's recovery and speedy return to the work team. Employees with considerable longevity feel slighted or offended when ignored during such a difficult time. Certainly no employer wants to give even the appearance of attempting to pressure an injured worker to return prematurely; however, care should be taken to avoid sending a message that the worker is not wanted or appreciated.

Return to work, even after healing has occurred, may continue to expose workers to further job site risks that brought about the initial injury. If a pattern of low back pain is identified in a particular job assignment, an evaluation should be performed to determine whether or not job site modifications are needed.

It is critical to monitor possible disincentives for returning to work. Those who seek or plan to pursue support or benefits from a government entitlement program (such as Social Security Disability Insurance) are less likely to be receptive to job placement. Those plaintiffs who claim that "My doctor told me I would never work again" usually have distorted reality and systematic inquiry often will reveal that no such prediction was ever made. However, since perceptions are such a powerful influence on behavior, it is the utmost importance that during the discovery process the plaintiff's assumptions, perceptions and expectations be uncovered.

Many factors must be considered in predicting return to work. These include age, education, psychological adjustment, economic disincentives, transferable skills, ability to drive, work ethic and personal goals. Those with higher levels of job satisfaction are less likely to become litigious.

SUMMARY

In light of many recent trends throughout the U.S. in litigation, it is easy to overlook the fact that a large number of disabled persons are able to work at least part-time, which signifies that disability does not universally mean a lack of work capacity and employability. While most court proceedings mandate an "either/ or" outcome, that need not be the only parameters for defending parties to consider. When weighing the merits of a plaintiff's allegations, consider a range of the merits of a plaintiff's allegations, consider a range of options which includes the worker returning to his or her former job with the same company; worker ready for modified return to job with same employer; rehabilitation; transfer to a new company (in same or similar job); retraining; or Social Security Disability or long-term disability insurance benefits for the patient who is irrevocably disabled (last resort). Returning to the same employer, even if for lighter duty and lower pay, is generally preferable and less stressful for the individual. In some instances, referral to state vocational rehabilitation programs should be recommended.

A comprehensive file review by a qualified vocational consultant will frequently unearth the probability of which options are most likely to apply to a given plaintiff. More often, a thorough vocational and psychological assessment will generate the data needed to help defend against soft tissue injury allegations. During the course of tracking the outcome of allegedly disabled individuals, we find that some do succeed in returning to gainful employment.

Vocational consultants need to become closely acquainted with the recently enacted Americans with Disabilities Act (ADA). About 43 million Americans meet the criteria for being classified as disabled. From a defense standpoint, this legislation can be cited to advantage. That is, if the objectives of the legislation are met, then a level playing field for the disabled or handicapped job applicant will ultimately be created. If a reasonable accommodation by the employer is necessary for the disabled individual to perform the duties of the job, they must be provided. Of course, reasonable accommodation is a somewhat vague term parameters for which remain to be adjudicated.

Realistically, legislation in the past has not changed attitudes overnight. Consider civil rights, equal opportunity and affirmative action laws. They continue to be thwarted and undermined in some sectors. But in the long run, the ADA should assist disabled job applicants and society, too. An increasing number of vocational specialists are consulting to employers and helping them to understand how to deal with this legislation and to modify job descriptions and work stations to better suit the disabled worker and assist him/her to become productive in a safe work environment.

References

Anchor, K.N. (1994). Assessment of vocational disability: A follow-up survey of test instruments. *Advances in Medical Psychotherapy, 7,* 175-180.

Anchor, K.N. (1992). *Interdisciplinary Life Care Planning for Mentally and Physically Disabled Patients.* Athens, GA: Elliott and Fitzpatrick.

Anchor, K.N. (1991). *The Handbook of Medical Psychotherapy: Cost Effective Strategies in Mental Health.* Toronto, Canada: Hogrefe & Huber.

Anchor, K.N. & Pautler, T.G. (1993). *Theory and Practice of Medical Psychotherapy.* Dubuque, IA: Kendall/Hunt Publishing.

Kenneth N. Anchor, Ph.D., ABPP

Kenneth N. Anchor, Ph.D., ABPP, is Associate Professor of Psychology and Human Development at Vanderbilt University. His primary career interest is in the evaluation and treatment of disabled individuals. During his twenty-two years of practice as a vocational consultant, he has authored over eighty publications including two books and a manual on life care planning. He has lectured widely in Brazil, Hong Kong, Mexico and elsewhere. Dr. Anchor is a consultant to various governmental agencies including the Social Security Administration. He has taught courses on forensic psychology and has presented his research to various legal, rehabilitation, medical and mental health conferences. Dr. Anchor holds several board certifications and is a member of the National Association of Forensic Economists, the American Academy of Economic and Financial Expertise and the American Association of Spinal Cord Injury Psychologists. He is frequently called upon to testify in litigation based upon his extensive experience in having evaluated over six thousand individuals alleging disability.

5

CASE MANAGEMENT IN FORENSIC REHABILITATION

Heidi Fawber, M.Ed., CRC, CCM
Barbara Zorger Orstein, M.Ed., CRC, CCM

Forensic case management is a relatively new concept. This can be defined as when case management services are used for the purpose of legal case preparation. Forensic case management can be a valuable service to both plaintiff and defense attorney's alike. To further explore forensic case management, it is helpful to review the history of case management. Many of the fundamentals of case management help to define this new specialty in forensic rehabilitation.

Overview of Case Management

As an independent discipline, case management is still developing, gradually forming specialties, as have other disciplines in rehabilitation. In the 1960's vocational rehabilitation and case management were found to offer potential cost savings on worker's compensation cases in several ways: by reducing lost wages, by minimizing insurance premiums and by helping employers avoid the need to hire and train new employees. During the 1960's and 1970's these benefits lead to the emergence of the private rehabilitation industry, which used case management services to assist insurance carriers in controlling costs of disability claims such as worker's compensation, personal injury and long-term disability. Case management, with its three distinct and interrelated features of goal orientation, individualization and sequential service delivery (Matkin, 1985), was extremely effective in managing these types of disability cases.

Case management has become a part of many different systems in the fields of medicine and rehabilitation as well as in state and federal programs and services. Case managers are now found in both acute and post-acute rehabilitation programs, in which they typically coordinate the admission and discharge processes as well as the services provided during the client's stay in programs. A case manager fills the role of central organizer of a client's program and is familiar with the client's progress in the program, and thus can act as a convenient source of accurate current outside information for agencies, funding sources and family members. The case manager must understand legal and insurance concerns in order to provide necessary and relevant documentation. The case manager must also be an expert in community resources or be knowledgeable about professionals who are aware of community resources to facilitate smooth transitions at the time of discharge. Sometimes establishing joint or cooperative programming is the best method for assisting a client. This type of programming requires close coordination of services, which is often best provided by an external case manager. Even communication within programs in made easier by a case manager since this person can act as the central hub for information gathered from all of the professionals in the program.

Specifically in the field of traumatic brain injury, "case management programs are being developed to coordinate and integrate service components, monitor quality of care, allocate financial resources, and document outcomes." (Kreutzer, Zasler, Wehman & Devany, 1991)

Case managers can be independent consultants making their services available to the insurance industry, self-insured employers, attorneys, state worker's compensation systems and other state-run programs requiring disability case management. Case managers employed by private rehabilitation companies also serve these programs. Some state-funded programs, such as the Virginia Case

Management Program for Traumatic Brain Injury, use in-house case managers to coordinate and follow complex disability cases. The Pennsylvania Head Injury Program, developed by Pennsylvania's Department of Health, is another example in which a state-funded program contracts with independent case managers to coordinate its cases.

It is difficult to define case management in one comprehensive statement. Case management has been defined as "the combination of activities designed to insure appropriate use of medical care facilities, improve quality of care, control or reduce costs, insure proper referrals, provide primary care, and manage patient's episodes of care, disability and rehabilitation." (Hembree, 1985) While another definition of case management is "the organization and sequencing of services and resources to respond to an individual's health care problem." (Merrill, 1985). The best approach to defining case management may be to identify the many possible functions and/or roles of a case manager, as well as to define the process of case management itself.

The Case Management Process

That case management is an on-going, evaluative/re-evaluative process reflects the fact that it is a dynamic process rather than a specific intervention. The term "case management" obviously had its basis drawn from the concept of "management". It becomes interesting to note that "the managerial process consists of four functions that must be performed by every manager: planning, organizing, leading and controlling." (Boone & Kurtz, 1984) Henri Fayol, a French management theorist, is usually credited with these four basic functions of the managerial process. This readily translates into the field of case management and defines the case management process succinctly. Indeed, every case manager must follow these steps of planning, organizing, leading and controlling the work on every given case.

In an optimal scenario, the case manager first becomes involved at the onset of the injury or disability and follows the client throughout the treatment process to achievement of his or her maximal level of functioning. This establishes the case management process, so that planning and organizing activities can be initiated. Follow-along or monitoring of the case over the long term is often the most effective use of case management. Case management involvement at times may be very active; at other times only limited activity may be required. Normally long-term case management diminishes in intensity over time. Specific short-term intervention is a potential use of the case manager which is often seen in forensic cases. This function may be used to assist in preparing cases for litigation. Case management activities aimed at identifying specialized and appropriate services can be used to assess clients in preparing legal cases. Short-term case management may also be used during transitions between programs or at discharge from a program back to home to insure a smooth transition and initiation of home-based services.

Overview of Forensic Case Management

Case management is a relatively new discipline, and therefore it is still developing sub-specialties. One such sub-specialty is that of forensic case management. In forensic rehabilitation, the case manager is most likely to be contracted with to perform a specific service, which the attorney may feel unqualified to perform, due to lack of expertise, lack of time, or other reason related to the attorney's ability to prepare the case for litigation. Attorneys need to regard the case manager as one who is qualified to render an opinion. In the courts, a case manager may only offer an opinion, if the education and experience, i.e. the credentials, are considered "expert". This issue is crucial before the case manager even begins to work on a case. Case managers must always specialize in objectivity, not only with regard to the case, but also in reference to their own strengths and weaknesses.

In forensic rehabilitation, the case manager must be knowledgeable both in rehabilitation and the litigation process. Case managers need to understand legal terminology, as well as how a case moves through the legal process, in order to effectively perform their jobs. By being knowledgeable in the forensic realm, the case manager may even consult on case strategy.

Case managers must be able to maintain clear understanding of who the real client is: the represented individual or the attorney who has obtained the case management services. Objectivity is essential on the part of the case manager. It is important in the forensics practice that the case manager not become an "over-advocate", thus losing sight of the original purpose for which services were retained. Recognition for which side of the court they have been retained, plaintiff or defense, is essential. It is clear that if a case manager is providing plaintiff services, then the attorney is looking for top dollar recommendations. While attorneys are typically pleased with a conservative approach, the higher the costs projected, the greater the chance for a higher reward. On the other hand, the goal for the attorney for the defense is the opposite. "Give them what they need, but no more" is the common philosophy.

The Roles of Case Managers

• Case management is often defined by the role the case manager is hired for and the functions that the role dictates. Case managers function in one or more of the following roles:

- *Advocate* - insuring that the client's needs are being met and rights are not compromised;
- *Facilitator* - insuring that services are identified, accessed, initiated and provided in a smooth fashion;
- *Coordinator* - interfacing with all pertinent parties in the case including client, family members, attorney, funding source, employer, school officials and health-care professionals; insuring prompt, cost-effective and well-planned service delivery;
- *Educator* - teaching family members and other professionals about a disability, its effects and the services needed to

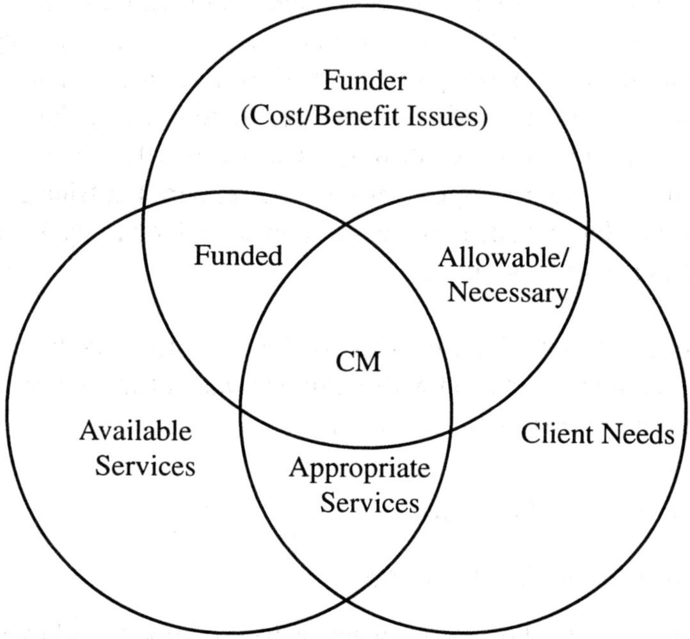

FIGURE 5.1 *The Integral Role of Case Management in the Rehabilitation Arena*

manage it; justifying and providing a rationale for the use of programs and services to funding sources; assisting legal professionals in preparing cases for trial or teaching juries about disabilities and their long-term effects;

- *Problem solver* - acting quickly as a "front-line" professional (often the case manager is the only professional involved in the case in a position to do so) to resolve problems which, due to unforeseeable or unavoidable circumstances, arise despite attempts to develop proactive plans;
- *Cost containment specialist* - acting as liaison between funding sources and clients to balance the need for service and the cost effectiveness of the service; monitoring services

to insure that clients achieve therapeutic gain as a result of services; planning and organizing service delivery to maximize benefit gained per dollar spent; identifying appropriate and effective services to help insure that funds are spent wisely. According to Calogero (1990, p. 25), who studied case management services rendered at Blue Cross/ Blue Shield, approximately $11 are saved for every $1 spent on case management.

The interactions of these facets of the case management role both among themselves and within dimensions of the environment and client are depicted in Figure 5.1.

Case Management Functions

Implementor of the Life Care Plan

One function of the case manager is to implement and oversee the life care plan. As described in chapters two and seven, the life care plan provides a detailed analysis of all of the future services and supplies which will be required by an individual as a result of an injury or disability. Normally case management services are built into the plan to insure that included services are actually received by the client. The case manager locates the needed services, coordinates the initiation of services, monitors their delivery, identifies problems and intervenes as necessary. In short, the case manager actually acts as the supervisor of the life care plan. Often plans are prepared by someone other than the case manager and may provide several options for needed programs and services rather than specifically naming service providers. The case manager then identifies the specific and most appropriate services and service providers in collaboration with clients and family members.

Broker of Services

Cervelli (1990, p. 471) states that "case management is a strategy for guidance of the dynamic interactive elements of a care system. To be successful in this role the case manager must have authority to drive the system. This may come from administrative policies and agreements between service agencies, legal and legislative mandates, fiscal control and responsibility, and clinical expertise." Authority must be delegated to the case manager in order for him or her to truly manage a forensic case. Appropriate services are carefully selected by the case manager and expectations for potential treatment outcomes are discussed with the service provider. Specific cost projections are clarified prior to the client's initiating the program or service. At times the experienced case manager may be able to negotiate special rates for a specific case when he or she is given the authority to make the decision to refer for services. Much of the ability of the case manager to function effectively as a broker of services is dependent on the degree of control delegated by the referral source.

Collateral Source Advisor

Upon a client's discharge from a hospital or other treatment program, publicly-funded programs may offer services known in the legal arena as collateral source programs. With regard to such programs it is important for the case manager to be aware that if the client is involved in litigation, the attorney must follow certain rules regarding notification and/or paybacks. These rules, unless federal programs such as Medicare or Supplemental Security Income are involved, vary from state to state. The case manager must also be aware that these programs cannot be presented in most courts as future service providers due to possible program rule changes which might occur; the only guaranteed program is Public Law 101-476, which provides for education and associated services for disabled children. Other programs are not guaranteed and can change based on funding streams, timing relative to fiscal years, as well as admission criteria. Lastly, many programs are typically dependent on funding availability as well.

On-site Coordinator

One dynamic of case management which has great bearing on its effectiveness and flexibility is that most case managers perform their jobs "in the field." They are generally very mobile as they attempt to personally assess situations, placements, programs and individuals. It is often very important to visualize a situation to best ascertain benefits, needs and potential problems with placements. Meeting with the client and family in person, at their homes or in their communities, significantly enhances the case manager's ability to gather pertinent information. Interventions and problem solving are often much more effective and efficient when they occur in the community than when they take place in a location separate from the community, such as a rehabilitation facility. This on-site involvement in cases often is not possible for other professionals due to the limitations of their roles. The case manager's personal access to the case enables him or her to communicate information to the other parties involved in the case and thereby facilitate their case intervention as well. In areas where limited specialized rehabilitative programs are available, there is no greater resource than a creative case manager. Often individualized programs must be "created" out of existing services which may not be fully appropriate unless modified in some way. In rural areas clients may be sent far from their homes for specialized rehabilitative programming; then, when discharge time draws near or funding has been exhausted, a return to home must be considered. Lack of services, transportation and awareness are common problems encountered when a client returns to a rural area. The case manager's role is to identify what is available and to attempt to develop a service delivery system out of existing local resources. To accomplish this, the case manager must act both as educator and coordinator. An example of this dual role is provided by the case of an 18-year-old traumatically brain injured young man who was returned from an out-of-state treatment facility to his home in a rural, sparsely-populated state. No outpatient brain injury services were available in the client's local area; therefore, during the summer months a special education teacher was hired to provide individualized programming for him following the individualized education plan devised during the previous school year ultimately preventing regression during the summer months.

In forensic rehabilitation this creative/innovative service development type of case management can be very useful. Identification of resources and services available in remote locations is essential for effective planning. Often effective networking with existing program staff yields valuable information for future planning. A working knowledge of a wide array of rehabilitation programs can assist the case manager in evaluating existing programs which might be used for a given case, with or without modification.

Case Management Providers

Those who perform case management are referred to by designations dependent on their training and background as well as by job titles. Some of these titles include rehabilitation counselor, rehabilitation coordinator, rehabilitation consultant and case manager. Many individuals holding these titles have completed training in rehabilitation counseling or a related field such as psychology or education. They tend to follow a vocational rehabilitation educational track and work in public agencies such as state vocational rehabilitation agencies or not-for-profit agencies that assist individuals with job training or job placement.

Those following a more clinical or medically-oriented educational track possess some similarities in day-to-day function, although their training and credentials are somewhat different from those of case managers following a vocational rehabilitation track. Rehabilitation nurse, rehabilitation consultant and case manager are titles held by nurses in the rehabilitation field; these professionals are found in rehabilitation hospitals, private rehabilitation companies, home health agencies, or in private practice as consultants.

In addition to working in the public sector, all types of rehabilitation professionals are frequently self-employed or employed by private-sector firms. Many case managers, particularly in the forensic sub-specialty are independent contractors. This may enhance their objectivity to some extent and may permit some additional freedom/independence to perform the complex array of job duties. Kaufman and Lichtenstein state that "case managers are most beneficial during initial transition from hospital to home. This is most true when the case manager is an independent practitioner whose only job is case management." (1990, p. 12) An independent case manager's effectiveness results in large measure from the independence of his or her decisions from control by funding sources.

CASE MANAGEMENT ACTIVITIES

The process of case management defines the functions encompassed by it. Not only are rehabilitation specialists routinely used by the insurance industry to move cases to closure, but the legal profession is beginning to use them to expedite case movement through the legal process. Forensic case management includes activities that are carried out on an ongoing basis. These include:

- *Assessment.* The case manager must assess the needs of the client and sometimes of the family. Careful consideration in conducting this assessment must be given to expectations of the individual and family as well as to their socioeconomic, cultural and religious backgrounds. In addition, the age of the individual along with any unique problems to be addressed must be included in any assessment. A comprehensive assessment includes a detailed premorbid history and a detailed account of the current status of the client. A formal interview is conducted and assessment or diagnostic tools are applied during the assessment phase.

- *Analysis.* Following the assessment phase, the case manager analyzes the information prior to making recommendations. Some questions to be answered at this stage are: What services will benefit the client? Will the funder pay for these services? Who is responsible for funding the services? Are the services a means for achieving rehabilitation goals or are they just an answer to whims of the client or family members? Do they satisfy the purpose for which the case manager was retained?

- *Service procurement.* Following identification of the client's needs, services must be located to meet these needs. Consideration must be given to costs, location, appropriateness of treatment or services, accessibility of services, admission criteria and potential outcome.

- *Referral.* The case manager is in a unique position to refer a client to an array of services; this does not infer that the client/family is not part of the decision-making process, but assumes that a decision has already been made. The case manager typically has all essential referral information at hand at this stage, if a complete assessment has been done.

- *Negotiation.* The case manager may be able to negotiate rates. This ability is especially helpful when the final amount of funding available has not yet been determined. For example, if an attorney is willing to guarantee payment through a letter of protection, it behooves the case manager to negotiate a rate since the cost of the service ultimately will be paid by the client (not at an insurance company's rate) out of proceeds from an award.

- *Education.* An important responsibility of the case manager is to educate all parties about the issues involved in the case. This task may mean educating an attorney about an unusual disability and its implications; it may mean educating an insurance company about a unique treatment available for a client; it may mean educating the family as to what are realistic expectations for their loved one.

Educating is especially important in the legal arena. If the case manager cannot help others to understand the needs of a disabled person, how will the case manager educate the opposing side or the jury? This issue represents a real concern of attorneys who hire case managers for case preparation, and should be a major concern of case managers who choose to work in forensic rehabilitation.

- *Documentation.* Concise documentation of dates, contacts and outcomes must be maintained for each case. It is advisable to include telephone numbers in case documentation, especially if the case manager initiates contacts. This information is essential to define the work performed on the case.

  Reporting should contain proactive rehabilitation recommendations which can be defended if necessary. Signature of the report's preparer should appear on each report so that there is no question as to who performed the activities being reported or who prepared the report.

- *Coordination.* The case manager's coordination of an individual's treatment insures that fragmentation and duplication of services are minimized, which is important in achieving what is best for the individual client and for case progress. Duplication of services may lead the opposing side to assume that the individual is building the case financially to obtain a larger award; fragmentation leads to mismanagement of cases and may create the impression that the client is "doctor shopping" and trying to build the case to increase the financial award. A very important function of the case manager is to eliminate these two problems. The client ultimately is the chief beneficiary of effective case coordination.

- *Advocating.* A case manager must be able to advocate for the client, including taking a stand which may be negatively perceived by the insurance company, the attorney or even the client's family. Advocacy may require helping to create a program not yet in existence. It may mean locating alternative funding sources. Ultimately advocating requires that the case manager is committed to the recommendations and will not back down in the face of fear of case closure. Being prepared to defend the recommendations made is primary. If the client has a need, the case manager must "sell" it.

- *Monitoring.* When a client is in a treatment program, the case manager's role is to monitor the treatment. Monitoring is not passive, rather it requires taking an active role in the treatment process and with the provider's treatment team. It means asking questions, planning ahead, looking beyond discharge; it means assisting with realistic goal setting by program staff; it means having a clear understanding of treatment goals and insuring that these goals are met.

- *Building linkages.* Linkages are essential to the ongoing case management process. Frequently the case manager is that link between a service provider and the family, the insurer, the attorney and other facilities or service providers. It is important to keep channels of communication open to smooth transitions, facilitate understanding of goals, and insure that treatment goals and attorney case development are realistic.

The active processes of case management include: assessment, organizing, coordinating, referring, negotiating, counseling and reassessing. He describes this as following a sequential pattern with some of the processes occurring simultaneously and/or repeated frequently (Dixon, 1989).

Benefits of Case Management

To the Client

The case manager is the client's ally who provides support and understanding in an often confusing medical/legal arena. As advocate the case manager attempts to insure that clients have access to all of the information and resources needed to make informed decisions. Empowering clients is one responsibility of the case manager and may involve coordination with an assigned advocate at times when clients are unable to advocate for themselves. Working together with clients can often help prevent problems from developing, especially during periods of transition. For example, upon discharge from a program, clients and their families are usually briefed by the provider's staff on treatment recommendations, which can be an overwhelming experience. The case manager can often simplify a complex maze of programs, services and funding issues for the client and smooth transitions back to school, work or other treatment programs.

Clients benefit from case management through increased income, enhanced societal expectations and acceptance, improved social and familial relationships, and psychological functioning. Educating the family, friends and others involved in the client's situation (teachers, employers and others) regarding the ramifications of disabling conditions can avoid misunderstanding or stigma. Acting as a buffer or running interference, also a function of case management, can assist clients to avoid direct confrontation with problems which they are not equipped to handle.

As allies or partners in the rehabilitation process, clients may be more willing to accept recommendations for services or treatments from the case manager than from others such as family members or facility professionals, thereby increasing client cooperation with seeking necessary services.

Substance abuse is frequently a problem for disabled individuals and needs to be addressed promptly. Often case managers can identify the existence of problems such as substance abuse due to their access to clients within the community environment.

Maintaining open lines of communication with clients and the many other parties involved in cases is a key benefit of case management intervention in situations such as this.

To the Family

The benefits of case management are also frequently experienced by the family. Case management must recognize the significant impact that a family can have on the case and must therefore include the "family" when appropriate. According to Kaufman and Lichtenstein, "the concept of what constitutes a family differs from culture to culture, and perhaps no appropriate words exist to indicate the diversity of arrangements that characterize the traditional family. Whatever the family constellation, family centered and culturally sensitive case managers support and assist families in their natural role as the primary caretakers of their children. The families must be equal partners with professionals, and collaborate in all aspects of decision-making with respect to provision of services . . . for their children." (1990, p.13)

Accommodations must be made when working with single-parent families. Issues relating to religious and cultural backgrounds and to socioeconomic status must also be recognized. For example, a Mennonite or Amish family may not have insurance benefits or be interested in pursuing state or federal programs.

To the Service Provider

Independent case managers can function as part of treatment facilities' teams. Being made aware of home-based or community-based issues which affect the client can be very useful to the treatment team and facilitate pre-discharge planning. The case manager's knowledge of community resources can help enable the team to provide appropriate programming in preparation for discharging the client back to the community. Information about resources available to the client in the home and community can be valuable to service providers and can increase the effectiveness of referrals to other providers.

To the Employer

Case management benefits employers in four ways: by stabilizing insurance premiums, by enhancing benefit packages, by improving human resource utilization (for instance, by reducing employee turnover and absenteeism) and by contributing to efforts to increase corporate social responsibility (Matkin, 1985). Cost savings are a direct benefit of case management services. Appropriate referral for needed services, careful monitoring and direct intervention when necessary, all areas in which case managers have expertise, also provide fiscal and human resource benefits for employers. As advocates case managers can act as aids and resources for employees. Case management therefore provides a dual benefit for employers, helping to control costs and manage the direction of a case and helping to humanize a complex disability system.

To the Insurance Carrier

Case management helps insurance carriers by:

- reducing liability by eliminating or reducing benefit payments;
- stabilizing reserve funds;
- minimizing duration of disability and/or medical costs, thus reducing loss ratios and keeping premiums stable;
- lessening the effects of disability;
- enhancing market competitiveness;
- increasing corporate social responsibility. (Matkin, 1985)

Insurance carriers frequently use forensic case management for worker's compensation cases. Many of these cases require specialization in vocational rehabilitation to assess a client's ability to work and perform jobs in order to determine whether the client will continue to receive benefits. A thorough and accurate work-up of the case is essential for this type of case preparation and can become a concise testimony presentation which displays the work which has been completed. Later, this case documentation can become an exhibit for the defense and can be entered as evidence.

Testimony may be regarded by the court as factual or expert. In order to be ruled as an expert witness, the case manager must have reasonable training, knowledge and experience in the rehabilitation/vocational field. If the case manager is not ruled an expert, only facts from his or her testimony may be accepted as evidence. Case managers are not allowed to render opinions unless they are accepted as expert witnesses. Clearly case managers can be assets to insurance carriers if they are regarded as experts.

Insurers other than worker's compensation carriers utilize case managers for peer reviews, resolving questions of medical necessity and determining the reasonableness of costs for care and services. Thus, the case manager has many ways of benefiting the insurance industry.

To the Attorney

While insurance carriers may be the primary funders of services, attorneys can also become funders through letters of protection. These letters are frequently issued when there is no obvious funding for a service, liability is clear and there is substantial assurance that the proceeds from the case will ultimately pay for a service. Rehabilitation facilities or other large providers may be willing to consider letters of protection as adequate assurance of compensation for services rendered, but independent contractors such as therapists or psychologists may not be in a financial position to wait the months or years for payment often necessary with letters of protection.

Case managers can explore with facilities their willingness to consider letters of protection when treatment is essential and delaying the onset of treatment may be detrimental to the client. If the facility agrees to initiate treatment, the attorney is responsible for completing the necessary paperwork.

Case management may also be part of case preparation. For the plaintiff attorney all of the functions outlined above can be performed as an ongoing process: records may be reviewed and summarized; recommendations for evaluations to assist with case development may be needed; a report outlining the client's medical history, current status and physical, emotional and social functioning may also be required to solidify the case.

Defense attorneys may find case managers useful for reviewing and summarizing records; arranging independent evaluations; obtaining experts (such as independent medical examiners, treating physicians, vocational experts, or economists, to name a few) for opinions on disability, liability or treatment issues; and reviewing opposing reports. Attorneys find that there is a growing need for these functions, particularly for cases involving unusual disabilities or catastrophic injuries and for clients having extensive treatment resulting in voluminous and sometimes confusing records. A case manager can clarify these matters and make recommendations in accordance with them.

Case managers may also be used by attorneys to assist in addressing legal guardianship or power of attorney issues. A case manager who has direct knowledge of a client and the proposed guardian can testify as to the benefits of a specific guardian or advocate for removal of a guardian for reasons such as abuse or medical neglect.

Case Management's Relationship to the Referral Source

When an attorney refers a case, there is frequently confusion as to what is needed or expected by the case manager. At the time of referral the medical records should be provided to the case manager together with a clear statement of what services the case manager is being asked to provide. A specific and precise statement of the request avoids later perceptions by the attorney of a case manager's having mismanaged the case.

Many case managers request a retainer for services to defray initial costs and guarantee that there is at least some payment for services rendered. Billing can occur monthly or following completion of work. Clear expectations about costs and services to be provided by the case manager will promote a positive working relationship with the attorney and avoid problems related to the case manager's bill.

Some attorneys are not completely comfortable with allowing case managers to make referrals directly to other professionals. Attorneys are knowledgeable of other experts' ability to testify in the court. The attorney may have knowledge about another professional's credentials. Often a case manager may not be aware of this type of information concerning other professionals. The attorney may not want the other side to be aware of the case manager's involvement at the onset of the case. It is imperative that the case manager have a clear understanding of what the extent of their involvement will be on a given case. Otherwise, there is a great potential for problems to arise in the middle of the case. To avoid this kind of problem, identification of the direction of the case, setting goals for the case manager's involvement and specification of the attorney's goal in case preparation must be conducted as a collaborative process.

When the referral is made by an insurance company, the goals are usually well defined by the type of claim. Nevertheless, clear delineation of the role and level of responsibility of the case manager is important in this type of case as well. It is important that the case manager act as the expert on the case in order to maintain control over the direction of the case.

Families are beginning to employ case managers to assist with the implementation of life care plans. In this situation, the family contracts with the case manager directly. The case manager delineates his or her level of involvement, the cost of case management services and the duration of the services so that there is a clear understanding with the family regarding expectations. This step is essential despite the fact that the life care plan may have already outlined these factors in order to maintain a positive working relationship between the case manager and the family.

PROFESSIONALISM

Ethical Issues

What happens when the client is an adult and has a legal guardian whose goals are clearly in opposition to the client's goals and when the case manager is in closer agreement with the client than with the guardian?

What happens when a facility obtains a contract to provide external case management with the goal of utilizing it as an indirect method of receiving referrals for in-house treatment?

What happens when the case manager is directed to prepare a report outlining a brain-damaged client's functioning when there has been no neuropsychological evaluation and when there is no funding for such an evaluation? Does the case manager still prepare a report?

Should a case manager accept gifts or remuneration for a referral?

The case manager finds a creative way to fund a service; there is a fine line between creativity and fraud. How should the case manager proceed?

The case manager is asked for a curriculum vitae. The case manager is not yet certified, but knows he will be within several months. He lists himself as being certified anyway.

Should a case manager work for an attorney who has questionable ethics according to the legal community at large? These situations define some areas which may present ethical issues. Some are dilemmas of conscience, while others are clear violations of codes of conduct or conflicts of interest.

Rehabilitation professionals need to concern themselves with ethical issues such as these. Basing choices regarding one's conduct not only on what is legal but on what is moral and ethical enables one to keep a clear focus on his or her own ethical position. Other professionals (not necessarily co-workers) can act as sounding boards or advisors to assist one in making sound ethical decisions and avoiding the pitfalls of conflicts and lack of professionalism.

Challenges to the Profession

Four primary challenges to professionalism in case management are expertise, certification, accountability and malpractice.

- Expertise is perhaps the most critical and least quantifiable qualities of case managers especially in forensic case management. Without expertise a case manager cannot take the proactive and visionary approach vital to effective case management.

  Expertise is not comprised of the training and education of a case manager alone. Among others, experience is another important component; the amount of experience, its relevance, comprehensiveness and depth are important factors. Another major component is the ability to think on one's feet when cases unravel. Only with adequate expertise can the case manager react quickly, confidently and correctly in situations such as this.

  Once expertise has been developed it must be maintained. Serious participation in continuing education is essential for case managers' maintenance of their expertise as well as their status as expert witnesses in the eyes of the court.

- Certification is becoming an increasingly challenging issue in rehabilitation. The original Certified Rehabilitation Counselor designation was followed by Certified Insurance Rehabilitation Specialist. The most recent new classification is that of Certified Case Manager. There are additional designations for vocational experts, vocational evaluators rehabilitation nurses and other related professionals. For the case manager, the challenge is to determine which certification to pursue and whether there is a need to specialize and in which area. Maintaining the qualifications for multiple specialist certifications will potentially become a challenge.

- Malpractice is becoming a critical issue in rehabilitation as it has in other health-care fields. Declining availability of funding and our litigious society make it likely that the number of malpractice suits will grow and affect case managers as they do other rehabilitation professionals. The malpractice issue is of particular importance for forensic rehabilitation case managers. A case manager who breaches confidentiality, who violates the Americans with Disabilities Act, or who does not involve the client or family in decision making prior to a referral, program or service provider, may be at risk for a malpractice suit.

Accurate documentation of cases, training in state and federal laws and policies and a clear understanding of the legal rights of disabled persons will help case managers avoid potential malpractice lawsuits and protect themselves in the event that they are sued for malpractice. Individual liability or malpractice insurance is also advisable for case managers.

- Accountability has always been an important issue in rehabilitation. The highest level of accountability is required in forensic rehabilitation. Accountability requires insuring that case managers' work is highly professional, accurate, objective and credible at all times. Case managers' first responsibility is to their clients and after that to the professionals who have retained their services.

The Development of the Field of Forensic Case Management

By the title of this book alone it is clear that a major trend in rehabilitation is the growing importance of forensic rehabilitation. More and more rehabilitation professionals including case managers are being hired to provide expert testimony and other services related to legal work. Forensic case managers must always be prepared to defend their rehabilitation plans and practices before a court, whether on behalf of a client, the insured or themselves.

Case managers are beginning to specialize in fields such as neurological disorders, drug and alcohol problems, burn rehabilitation, AIDS and HIV infections and pediatric disabilities.

Increasing specialization is another trend which is beginning to affect forensic case management. All case managers cannot be specialists in every disabling condition. The rapid expansion of new laws, treatments, technologies and information will make it necessary for case managers to narrow their fields of expertise.

A trend related to the increasing specialization in rehabilitation is the growing demand for licensing and certification of rehabilitation professionals. As described earlier, there are many new specialty areas of certification. It is anticipated that there will continue to be more in the future. Most case managers choose to become certified in their areas of expertise. Licensure is also growing with 38 states having requirements affecting case management.

Conclusion

Case managers' roles are expanding in the 1990's, especially in the forensic environment. Case management is a tool which can be used to assist with case preparation, to identify resources and to provide assessments and documentation. It is rapidly becoming an integral part of the legal arena, particularly in cases involving personal injury, medical malpractice suits and worker's compensation.

Forensic case managers perform the functions of life care plan implementor, broker of services, collateral source advisor and on-site coordinator. Individuals providing forensic case management services are known by a variety of titles and may have various educational backgrounds. Their functions are, however, similar in the activities they perform: assessment, analysis, service procurement, referral, negotiation, education, documentation, coordination, advocating, monitoring and building linkages.

Forensic rehabilitation provides benefits to a wide circle of persons involved in the case, including the client and members of his or her family, service providers, employers, insurance carriers and attorneys.

Forensic case managers will emerge as a knowledgeable, well-trained and diverse group of professionals who, due to their professionalism, accountability and organizational and documentation skills, will become integral players of the forensic rehabilitation field.

Forensic case management will involve intrigue, high accountability, and the opportunity to work with legal professionals. It is a satisfying role which can be of great service to the represented client. Forensic case managers will have opportunities to participate in settlement negotiations, hearings and trials. It is not for the meek or unprepared case manager.

REFERENCES

Boone, L.E. & Kurtz, D.L. (1984). *Principles of Management.* Second edition. New York, NY: Random House.

Calogero, M.A. (1990). Individual case management and the Blue Cross and Blue Shield system. *The Case Manager,* Jan. Feb. March.

Cervelli, L. (1990). Re-Entry into the community with traumatic brain injury. In Rosenthal, M., et al, (Eds.). *Rehabilitation of the Adult and Child with Traumatic Brain Injury.* Philadelphia, PA: F.A. Davis Company.

Dixon, T.P. (1989). Systems of care for the head-injured. In L.J. Horn & D.N. Cope (Eds.) *Physical Medicine And Rehabilitation: State of the Art Reviews,* 3, 1. Philadelphia, PA: Hanley & Belfus, Inc.

Hembree, W.E. (1985). Getting involved: Employees as case managers. *Business and Health,* July/August, 11-14.

Kaufman, J. & Lichtenstein, K.A. (1990). Children with catastrophic illness: Principles of care management. *The Case Manager.* Oct. Nov. Dec.

Kreutzer, J.S., Zasler, N.D., Wehman, P.H., & Devany, C.W. (1991). Neuromedical and psychosocial aspects of rehabilitation after traumatic brain injury. In Fletcher, Jann, Wolf, & Banja (Eds.). *Rehabilitation Medicine: State of the Art.* Lea and Febier.

Matkin, R.E. (1985). *Insurance Rehabilitation.* Austin, TX: Pro-Ed.

Merrill, J.C. (1985). Defining case management. *Business and Health,* July/August.

Heidi L. Fawber, M.Ed., CRC, CCM

Ms. Fawber is a masters level rehabilitation counselor and is certified as both a rehabilitation counselor and case manager. She began her career in the rehabilitation field over 16 years ago, initially specializing in case management and vocational rehabilitation. By 1981, Ms. Fawber helped to create one of the country's first community re-entry programs for traumatically brain injured adults in Pittsburgh, PA. This program maximized case management services to attain successful case outcomes. She has authored several articles on this subject, as well as a chapter in the book Community Re-Entry for Head Injured Adults (Ylvisaker and Gobble, eds.). Since 1988, Ms. Fawber has been a private rehabilitation consultant, providing case management, life care planning and vocational expert services. This forensic practice has been centered in Pennsylvania and West Virginia. Ms. Fawber is currently the Program Coordinator - Outpatient Head Injury Services at Harmarville Rehabilitation Center in Pittsburgh. There she is developing a mild brain injury program, while continuing to provide forensic services.

Barbara Zorger Orstein, M.Ed., CRC, CCM

Ms. Orstein is a certified rehabilitation counselor and case manager. She has been in the field of rehabilitation for 14 years. She has a private forensic consulting practice in Harrisonburg, Pennsylvania. Ms. Orstein provides case management, life care planning and vocational expert services to attorneys. Her practice covers the Mid-Atlantic region with the majority of her referral base in the central Pennsylvania region.

6

ANALYSIS AND MANAGEMENT OF MILD HEAD INJURY

Bruce L. Bird, Ph.D.

Introduction

The terms "mild head injury" and "minor head injury" have been used to describe a wide range of neurobehavioral disorders with diverse pathologies and sequelae, based on initial presentation of cases and the capability of current medical practice to diagnose serious pathology. The terms "mild" and "minor" head injury can be very misleading. For a small percentage of patients, the pathologies and neurobehavioral sequelae are severe. For another substantial percentage, they are less "severe" as traditionally defined in neurorehabilitation, but severe in the physical and neurobehavioral sequelae which disrupt normal life. The vast majority of patients "fully" recover, with little or no obvious signs of sequelae.

Clinical and medi-legal decisions about "mild head injury" are fraught with peril. This chapter reviews the current literature, identifies problems in diagnostics and treatment, and attempts to provide guidance for professionals involved in case management, treatment, or medi-legal decisions in cases of mild head injury. It also identifies needs for further development in basic understanding and clinical practice in this controversial and developing area.

Case Study

Bob, a young man in his twenties, was referred to a community re-entry brain injury rehabilitation center by a very motivated employer, who wished to determine Bob's ability to return to work. After drinking heavily with friends, Bob attempted to get into his locked apartment by climbing balconies, and fell three stories to the ground. In his fall, he sustained a broken femur, bruised shoulder, and a "mild" head injury.

The head injury was "mild" because there was either no loss or a momentary loss of consciousness, and no other signs of severe neurologic damage. Dazed, slightly confused, but also with no post-traumatic amnesia, and intoxicated in the emergency room, Bob was admitted to the hospital to recover from his broken femur and for observation of his neurologic status. In a few days, Bob's confusion resolved. A neuropsychological examination was conducted to determine the extent of any residual cognitive deficits. The neuropsychological evaluation found mild but selected deficits in spatial memory (the ability to remember new information about spatial organization, locations, or maps), and mild problems in the executive functions of attending and concentrating. The employer was concerned that these cognitive deficits, plus a history of alcohol abuse, would adversely impact job performance. Both the employer and job were unusual, because of the training investment in Bob and the risks of the job. The employer was a branch of the U.S. Armed Forces and Bob's position was that of a flight line mechanic for the most advanced jet fighters in the world.

Over a six week period, Bob received evaluation and "treatment", returned to work, and experienced success on the job and in his personal life which was sustained at a six month follow-up. The key elements of rehabilitation were: Bob's acceptance of his cognitive limitations and substance abuse problems, and his motivation to work on these issues; the development of sufficiently detailed but non-burdensome compensatory strategies developed to assist him in his work (by speech/language and vocational specialists who went to the flight line to thoroughly assess his job and level of possible supervisory support); his employer's willingness to include special monitoring of Bob's compensatory strategies; his participation in AA and control of his alcohol problem.

The unanswerable question in this case is what would have happened had Bob not received help. Would he have adjusted with the help of friends and colleagues, or failed at his job and experienced personal problems in alcoholism, loss of unemployment, and perhaps worse?

Case management, treatment, and legal decisions about cases such as Bob's are extremely challenging. This chapter reviews current state of the art knowledge and practice in diagnosing mild head injuries, and outlines cautions and recommendations for medilegal and case management practitioners in this challenging area.

Demographics

The demographic evidence regarding outcomes of "mild" head injuries is very poor. The overwhelming majority of children and adults who have concussions or "mild" head injuries sufficiently serious to seek medical evaluation, recover and have little or no sequelae. A small but significant number, estimated as high as 20% of those experiencing injuries (NHIF, 1991) do not recover, and have residual problems in cognitive and behavioral functioning which range from mild to devastating. These unfortunate victims are certainly misclassified as having "mild" head injuries. Unlike the improving data base for individuals with severe traumatic brain injuries, the U.S. Health Care System provides very poor information on identification, treatment, and prognosis for cases of mild head injury.

Estimated incidences of mild head injury vary significantly. The National Head Injury Foundation (NHIF) has reported that about 325,000 people in the U.S. experience mild head injury each year. Anderson and McLaurin (1980) reported that of about 400,000 mild traumatic brain injuries (MTBI's) each year, about 20% had persistent adverse symptoms at 90 days. Levin and Eisenberg (1988) have reported that while the incidence of hospitalizations for all head injury is about 200/100,000 population, mild head injury accounts for about 2/3 to 3/4 of these admissions, and about 5 outpatients receive medical attention for head injury for every hospital admission.

Estimates of true incidence vary for several reasons. One is the varying definitions used by professionals and medical systems for diagnosing and treating mild head injury. Issues of definition and diagnosis are thoroughly reviewed in subsequent sections of this paper.

A second and related problem is the lack of mechanisms or systems for collecting and organizing data on mild head injury. The NIH Traumatic Coma Data Bank represents a major multi-center effort in standardizing diagnoses and organizing and analyzing incidences, types, clinical courses, sequelae, and "outcomes" of severe head injuries (Marshal et al., 1992). No such effort exists for the problems of "mild head injury".

A third problem is that people suffering from sequelae of mild head injury often seek services in the health care system which do not recognize the presenting symptoms as sequela of traumatic brain injury. If these services do accurately diagnose the underlying pathology, they do not organize or contribute to service data on incidences of mild head injury. For example, patients presenting with headache after mild head injury often present to psychiatry, neurology, or pain management services, where they may be diagnosed as migraine sufferers and treated inappropriately. Neuropsychiatric symptoms of depression often lead the patient to present to psychiatry services where, even if appropriately diagnosed and treated, it is rare that such incidences are aggregated with other data on "mild head injuries" in the same service system (hospital, HMO, etc.).

A fourth problem relates to emergency room (ER) screening and handouts given patients and families to detect symptoms of head injury. These are designed to identify signs of severe, potentially life threatening brain injury, and usually do not identify possible sequelae of mild head injury. This issue will be reviewed in detail in a subsequent section of this chapter. For purposes of demographic data systems, current ER systems often are not helpful.

Obviously improvements in public awareness, medical education, and particularly increased alertness in ER, neurology, psychiatry, and psychology practitioners to screen for and assist in data collection, are all needed to improve information on mild head injury demographics.

Definitions

Traditional research literature and clinical practice classify head injuries into categories of "mild", "moderate", and "severe", based on a limited number of diagnostic procedures.

One criteria is the total duration of loss of consciousness. Mild head injuries are generally defined as a loss of consciousness of 30 minutes or less, or 20 minutes or less, depending upon the author and source (Levin & Eisenberg, 1988).

A second criteria is the Glasgow Coma Scale (GCS) rating "at the time of admission". In practice, the time of rating often varies, and in the literature there is growing awareness of the possible variance in predictive value of GCS at varying intervals as an individual patient experiences changes in symptoms and pathology over time (Levin, 1992).

Other criteria which are used include the presence and duration of post-traumatic amnesia, the presence/absence of other hard signs of pathology, such as skull fracture, detected hematoma or other neuropathological process, and the severity or persistence of significant symptoms of brain injury.

Table 6.1 depicts a simplistic scheme of definitions of head injury, based on key diagnostic criteria.

Table 6.2 depicts symptoms of brain injury by defined category, as frequently depicted in the literature.

Several issues are apparent in reviewing criteria for definitions. The first is that a "mild" head injury is not defined by the underlying neuropathology, except for exclusions of mass lesions, nor by the

TABLE 6.1 *Definitions of Mild, Moderate, Severe Head Injury*

	Severe	Moderate	Mild
Loss of Consciousness	30 minutes or greater	30 minutes to 24 hours	20 minutes or less
Glasgow Coma Scale	Below 8	8-12	13-15
Post Traumatic Amnesia	Prolonged	Prolonged	24 hours or less
CT or MRI	Positive	Positive	Negative for mass lesions
Neurologic Examinations	Positive	Positive	Normal or abnormal (slightly)
Complications/ Deterioration	Usually present	May be present	None

course of recovery of symptoms or pathological conditions.

The second issue concerns the value of the term "mild head injury" for indicating treatment or for predicting recoveries of neurobehavioral or cognitive functions. Without specifying the symptoms or underlying pathology in detail, predicting the timecourse and extent of recovery for an individual patient with "mild" head injury is practically impossible.

A third issue concerns symptoms clinicians and patients are trained to detect as indicators of an ongoing neurologic problem, and so, needed treatment. Trauma service staff are primarily focused on those disorders which require immediate life-saving intervention, and particularly patients who need hospitalization and/or surgical intervention (Tyson, 1988). This is appropriate, given their training and the resource priorities set in trauma care. Patients with "mild" head injuries are sent home with emergency room handouts and alerted to self-detect symptoms of severe neurological injury which indicate a need for hospitalization and treatment. These are also

TABLE 6.2 *Symptoms of Brain Injury*

	Severe	Moderate	Mild
Headache	+	+/-	+/-
Nausea	+ vomiting	+/-	+/-
Motor Skills	+	+/-	- or + slowed + dizziness
Speech - expressive	+ absent, slurred	+/-	-
Speech - receptive	+/-	+/-	- or + slowed
Attention	+/-	+/-	- or + distractible
Memory	+/-	+/-	- or + selective
Seizures	+/-	+/-	-
Emotional	+/-	+/-	- or + irritable + depressed + lability + anxiety
Sleep/activity	+	+/-	- or + disturbed - insomnia + fatigued
Executive functions	+/-	+/-	- or + disorganized + impulsive + can't do complex tasks
Sensory	+/-	+/-	- or + photophobia + noise - hypersensitivity
Resolution of problems	unresolved (many)	resolved or unresolved	resolved or unresolved

most appropriate practices, which often save lives as patients re-enter treatment systems as a result of neurological deterioration which may be life threatening. But, for a patient with a "mild" head injury who develops or continues with severe, persistent symptoms in neurobehavioral or cognitive areas, traditional emergency room screening/alert practices will not be helpful in guiding the patient back into care.

Because scientist/practitioners have recognized definitional problems and a lack of predictive value, use of the term "mild head injury" has been criticized. Zasler (1992) for example, has cogently argued for use of the term "acquired subtle brain injury", referring to the enduring neurologic/behavioral condition experienced by that small but significant percentage of individuals experiencing "mild head injury".

For the clinician, patient, or medi-legal practitioner, decisions about treatment and/or compensation must be made based on detailed reviews of diagnostic procedures, which indicate whether or not an individual has persistent neurologic, behavioral, cognitive, or other physical sequelae. In that regard, a "mild head injury" must be considered with the same seriousness as a "mild heart attack", as both have enduring impacts on an individual's life.

Mild head injuries do produce neuropathologies and sequelae which fall into several categories. In each category, the patient presents initially as having a "mild head injury", with the following criteria: GCS greater than 13, loss of consciousness of 30 minutes or less, and no other detectable neurological pathology (hematoma, etc.) Beyond this initial presentation, classifying the case into one of several major categories has critical impact on outcome.

One category defines the vast majority of patients who evidence no deterioration or developing neuropathology, over time, who exhibit no symptoms past a few hours or days, and who have a full recovery with no residual symptoms.

A second category might be considered as those who have more significant symptoms and complaints over a period of days or weeks, but who eventually return to a "full recovery". Typically these patients have complaints of "feeling bad", slowed information processing, headaches, and/or other selected physical, sensory, cognitive, or emotional/behavioral sequelae as listed in Table 6.1. Levin and Eisenberg (1988) have suggested that such mild head injured patients may be more susceptible to physical and behavioral stressors, and should consider taking two weeks of leave from productive activity such as work to recover. Again, the vast majority of these cases are reported to recover spontaneously to full lives over a period of about three months (Fisher, 1985).

A third category of cases are those who experience significant and serious physical, sensory, behavioral/emotional and/or cognitive sequelae long after the injury, and often permanently. Estimation of this population varies from 3 to 20% of the population of the total population of mild head injuries (Barth et al., 1983, Rimel et al., 1981, 1982) Because such cases often do not receive the benefits of new, more expensive diagnostic technologies, and because the relative accuracies of technologies of MRI's and SPECT's (discussed below) are as yet unproven, and certainly not generally accepted as needed for such cases, diagnoses and treatments for this population vary widely.

A fourth category of mild head injury cases develop severe, sometimes life-threatening pathologies and/or sequelae, due to active developing processes which may not be evident at initial screening or even for an initial period of observation and treatment lasting days. The relative proportion of cases in this category is small, estimated to be about 3% of the population (e.g., Dacey et al., 1986). However, they may require intensive immediate neurosurgical intervention to avoid coma, death, or permanent damage (Dacey et al., 1986). The literature is not consistent in categorizing cases in category 4 above as "mild head injuries", as the pathologies and sequelae are severe. That is, in a case initially presenting as "mild", once a clear severe pathology has been identified, the call is usually reclassified as "severe".

Finally, there are cases in which patients have clearly experienced an accident and a "mild head injury", in which they have physical (pain, usually), sensory, behavioral, and/or cognitive sequelae, who are experiencing post-traumatic stress disorder

(PTSD). PTSD has identifiable symptoms in the literature, which are significantly different from the sequelae of mild brain injury. Post traumatic stress disorder is defined by different symptoms, including: recurrent and persistent reexperiencing of the traumatic event; avoidance of thoughts, feelings, and/or situations associated with the event; apathy; loss of affect; high levels of anxiety; disturbed sleep cycle; hypervigilance. Differential diagnosis of PTSD is important, as treatment approaches are very different (Davidoff et al., 1988; Saigh, 1992).

For purposes of discussion in this chapter, "mild head injury" will be used to indicate the disorders indicated in categories 2 and 3 above. That is, those injuries which produce brain injury and neurological sequelae and symptoms which may be transient or permanent, but which produce disturbances of pain, sensation, cognition, and emotional/behavioral functions which are either severe but selective or, if pervasive, mild in intensity.

Before proceeding to review diagnostic and therapeutic technologies, the researcher and/or practitioner is well cautioned regarding additional issues of definition.

First, the key criteria which define mild head injury merit review. Whereas the reliability of the Glasgow Coma Scale (GCS) has been established as high in research studies involving a full range of severities of injuries, the reliabilities and validities of GCS's in practicing clinicians and especially in the high end of the range (13-15) may be rightfully questioned, as there is no available research on these particular topics. Estimates of the occurrence and/or duration of loss of consciousness in the literature are questionable, as eyewitnesses are often stressed and unreliable. Estimates of duration of post-traumatic amnesia have been reported in the literature as reasonably reliable when conducted by professionals in research settings. However, in practice, incidences of post-traumatic amnesia are often reported second-hand by untrained nonprofessionals, who provide less reliable data on their durations than those reported by professionals with modest amounts of training.

The literature on traumatic brain injury classifications has continued to develop finer analyses of classifications and definitions. For example, Colohan and Oyesikv (1992) have provided an insightful review of classifications of "moderate" head injury. They make cogent arguments for classifying two groups of patients, one with GCS of 9-10 in the first 8 hours of admission, and a second with GCS of 11-12, with a substantially higher proportions of cases who recover more fully on comprehensive disability ratings.

Proper identification of mildly vs. moderately injured patients is critical, given the well-supporter literature which indicates significant and severe debilitation of such patients on a number of measures, including psychosocial, adaptive living, and return-to-work indicators, which translate into significant financial losses and family burdens (Dikmen et al., 1993). Most studies of moderate and severely head injured individuals have found that more than half of those affected do not return to work (Schwab et al., 1993), and that a significant percentage of individuals with "moderate" injuries have severe quality of life disruptions (Klonoff et al, 1986).

Until a classification system based on improvements in neuroimaging and neurobehavioral observations is developed and becomes pervasive in practice, the definition problems noted will continue to plague researchers, practitioners, and medi-legal decision makers. Practitioners are therefore encouraged to question labels such as "mild" or "moderate" head injury, and to define the case by the symptoms and signs as assessed by diagnostic procedures.

Pathologies

The underlying neuropathology of an individual mild head injury may be any one of a number of disorders. By definition, as noted above, the more easily detected mass lesions, intracranial hematomas, or complications such as widespread anoxia, automatically classify the disorder as moderate or severe brain injury. A brief review of underlying pathologies and a more detailed review of diagnostic technologies follows.

Levin et al., 1989 have summarized the identified pathological bases for sequelae of mild head injury, as illustrated in Table 6.3. Of interest is that a majority of the pathologies listed are extracranial. The Levin and Eisenberg (1988) taxonomy also omits pathologies identified by other authors, including damage to intracerebral blood vessels proposed as the causes of trauma-induced migraines (Haas & Lourie, 1988).

TABLE 6.3 *Pathologies in Mild Head Injury*

Intracranial	• Mild diffuse axonal injury • Cerebral contusions (focal) • Intracranial hematomas (small) • Lesions in white matter (small) • Alteration of intracerebral vessels
Extracranial	• Labyrinth injuries • Scalp/cervical/upper torso, muscular, ligament, or spinal injuries • Superficial cranial vessels
Emotional	• Non-specific emotional truama • Life stressors due to accident/injuries
Pre-existing	• Pre-existing psychiatric, substance abuse, psychosocial, occupational disorders • Antecedent neurologic insults
Interactions	• Interactions of the above

(Expanded form Levin & Eisenberg, 1988)

Of the potential neuropathologies, the most commonly assumed in the clinical literatures are those which have also been verified by neuroimaging, particularly Magnetic Resonance Imaging (MRI) and Single Photon Emission Computerized Tomography (SPECT). These are Diffuse Axonal Injuries, contusions of frontal and temporal lobes, and small, sometimes microscopic shearing/tearing injuries of supporting non-neuronal tissue, and/or blood vessels. These injuries vary in severity and distribution throughout the brain, producing a range of brain injuries from mild to most severe. Corresponding sequelae vary from brief concussion syndrome in which the patient may be dazed, and/or experience brief reversible post and retrograde amnesia, to coma and/or death.

Diffuse Axonal Injury (DAI) refers to a condition in which neuronal axons are damaged by stretching and/or shearing. The physical structure of the brain is such that, if the brain is at rest, or moving, and is subjected to a quick or immediate change from acceleration to deceleration, or vice versa, not all structures stop or start at the same time, and the connections holding the brain together inside the skull stretch or tear. The connecting structures are nerves, and nerve axons, supporting cells, and blood vessels. Diffuse Axonal Injury has been demonstrated in animal models of head injury (Genarelli et al., 1982), in autopsies of patients with traumatic brain injuries (Blumberg et al., 1989), and in a growing number of studies of patients with severe, moderate, and even "mild" head injuries (Colohan & Oyesciku, 1992).

DAI can produce a brief period of disruption of neuronal communication, in the case of stretched axons, or permanent disruption of communication between brain areas, in the case of torn axons. Torn axons result in subsequent death of downstream neurons over a period of days/weeks. The extent and location of DAI depends on the velocity and location of impact. A number of authors have reviewed the range of disorders which may be produced by DAI (Blumberg et al., 1989). It is now believed that DAI is responsible for Post Traumatic Amnesia, which may occur as a result of stretching sensitive axons in the hippocampus, a brain area thought to be intimately involved in short term memory and conversion of short-term to long-term memory (Povlishock et al., 1992).

Severe brain injuries and death may result from greater forces exerted on long axons linking brain stem areas with other brain and spinal centers. Between a brief, reversible confusion and brain death lies a continuum of cognitive and neurologic disorders which may be produced by DAI. Genarelli et al., (1982a, b) and Adams et al., (1982) have studied the nature and extent of pathologies produced by acceleration/deceleration injuries in animals and patients with head injuries, and proposed categories for classifying diffuse brain injury primarily due to diffuse axonal injuries. These categories range from mild and reversible, attributed to cortical damage to severe, irreversible, attributed to brain stem damage. Although these findings are frequently referenced in the clinical literature, the classification system has no predictive or treatment-directive utility as adopted by the medical community.

The effects of less severe DAI, consisting of disorientation, confusions, and impaired attention, generally proposed to be due to diminished arousal of or isolation of frontal lobes (Saneda & Corrigan, 1992), are usually assumed, as these injuries are not detected by CT scans, nor usually by MRI's, although SPECT imaging has been more revealing, as discussed in detail below.

Contusions of frontal and temporal lobes have been cited as primary culprits in mild and moderate head injuries by many authors (Hart & Jacobs, 1993). The vulnerabilities of these areas are enhanced for two reasons - they are positioned against boney protrusions inside the skull, and most impacts in injuries often occur from the front or frontal quadrant.

Frontal and temporal lobe functions are among those which are most complex and most "human". The frontal lobes are involved in "executive" functions, which "decide what is worth attending to and what is worth doing", provide organization of behavior (requiring working memory, planning, sequencing of responses), modifies affective and social responses and drives, and is responsible for self-monitoring, self-awareness, and "metacognition", or thinking about thoughts and behavior (Hart & Jacobs, 1993). The frontal lobes are actually a system of subsystems which are highly complex and structured, and have been the subject of substantial clinical and basic research over the past twenty years (Stuss & Benson, 1986; Levin et al., 1991). Both global and selective frontal lobe dysfunctions have been identified with increasing clarity in developing neuropsychological assessments which evaluate such functions (Lezak, 1993). As discussed in more detail in the section on diagnostics, Magnetic Resonance Imaging (MRI) and newer but less available Single Photon Emission Computerized Tomography (SPECT) neuroimaging technologies have begun to develop correlational data confirming the relation between various types of frontal injuries and neurobehavioral sequela.

Of particular note has been the growing awareness that orbito-frontal (deep, lower medial frontal lobe) damage which produces anosmia, or loss of smell, is predictive of more severe disabilities in long term outcomes, even in patients who otherwise test normal on many psychological and neurological indicators (Varney & Menefee, 1993).

Haas and Lourie (1988) have reviewed the clinical research literature on transient trauma-induced migraine (TTM) headaches. Findings from their review conclude the following: the symptomatic expressions of TTM are identical to those of spontaneous migraines (ophthalmic distortions are common, severe pain, often localized to one hemisphere, nausea and vomiting, occasional motor weakness or hemiparesis occurs); patients with TTM often have spontaneous migraines; the incidences of spontaneous migraines in families of patients with TTM is higher than in the general population; angiograms, CT scans, EEG, and cerebrospinal fluid findings during TTM attacks are similar to those of spontaneous migraines.

The relationship of impact site to TTM incidence and presentation is unclear, as is the pathogenesis of TTM's. Susceptibility to traumatic spasm of cortical vessels or spreading depression of Leao (an electrochemical phenomena which can be experimentally produced in animals and could be due to cortical pressure against the skull) have been two proposed mechanisms for TTM. The potential role of muscular tension-induced migraines second to trauma has not been well discussed in the TTM literature, but has been implicated in classic migraines.

Zasler (1992) among others has cautioned clinicians about the potential overdiagnosis of head pain in patients with mild TBI as migraines. Pain perceived as intracranial may be referred from skeletomuscular problems in other areas of the head and neck. For example, pain "felt" at the vertex may be referred from the sternocleidomastoid muscles, at the occiptal area from the trapezius, and at the forehead from eye or frontalis muscles. Most importantly, muscular disorders such as myofascial pain disorders often respond positively to treatments such as nonsteroid antiinflammatories, relaxation training, TENS. Among the clinical features in TTM noted by Haas and Lurie (1988) are the time course of development of the migraine, which usually begins within 1 to 10 minutes of traumatic impact, but may be anywhere from 1 to 4 hours. Treatment for TTM includes analgesia and antiemetic agents for symptoms of pain and vomiting. Prophylactic use of medication and/or stress and muscle-tension reduction training, commonly used in treating classical migraines, have not been widely reported as used in this population, but would appear to have an appropriate role in TTM.

As will be reviewed in greater detail in the section on diagnostics, intracranial hematomas, white matter lesions, and vasomotor alterations of intracerebral blood vessels are detected only with difficulty, unless they are large, pervasive, and/or producing severe neurobehavioral sequelae. The location, nature, and extent of these injuries are related to the nature, location, and force of injury, but are also considered to be influenced by the individual anatomical "predisposition" of the individual. Extracranial injuries occur as a result of direct impact, or due to strains on ligaments, peripheral nerves and/or blood vessels due to rapid changes in force due to acceleration-deceleration accidents. Zasler (1992) has provided a most thorough review of the pathologies and differential diagnostics for these disorders.

Pathologies of emotional and psychiatric or psychosocial disorders may masquerade as or contribute to symptoms of neurobehavioral or cognitive deficiencies in mild head injuries. Because initial presenting symptoms may be similar, including headache, dizziness, attention disorders, or executive dysfunctions, differential diagnoses are needed which carefully assess pre-injury histories. Although not well researched or quantified, it is widely accepted among practitioners and researchers that the interactions of neurological injuries with emotional and psychosocial stressors and pathologies can produce devastating outcomes, even in mild head injury cases. Accordingly, treatments must address these interactions to be successful (Kay, 1986).

Outcomes

The current available literature on outcomes in mild and moderate head injury does not offer the clinical practitioner or medi-legal decision maker clear information to predict outcomes in a particular case (Barth et al., 1983; Rimel et al., 1981, 1982; Ruff, 1986; Rutherford, 1989). One reason is, as the next section indicates, diagnostic technologies are improving dramatically, but are still limited. A second is that this "disorder" is really a diverse array of disorders with correspondingly diverse pathologies, sequelae, and outcomes. Moreover, as indicated in the pathologies section above, the impact of social and emotional supports and stressors on the symptomatic expressions of neurological pathologies can be great. Such differences can produce two very different outcomes, measured in the individual's ability to function in the family or at work, in two patients with the same neurological problems. A third problem is that previous injuries or pre-existing psychiatric/psychological problems may be greatly exacerbated by a "mild" brain injury. These again can produce very different functional outcomes in patients with similar neuropathologies. Finally, outcome studies in the literature have struggled against substantial methodological problems, including the absence, limitation, or timing of diagnostics which adequately define neuropathologies and the attrition of subjects over a period of follow-up assessments. All of these factors have complicated interpretations of outcomes of "mild" head injury.

In a classic study, Rimel et al., (1981, 1982) found significant differences in predictors of unemployment for patients with mild and moderate head injuries. Socioeconomic and other demographic factors, including age, income, education, and level of employment were not predictive of return to employment for moderately injured patients, but were predictive for mildly injured patients. Overall, 69% of moderately injured patients gainfully employed pre-injury were unemployed post-injury, whereas only 34% gainfully employed prior to mild head injury were unemployed post-injury. Regarding symptomatic recoveries, 93% of moderately injured patients complained of headaches, 90% of memory deficits, and 4% were asymptomatic at 3 months. Using predictions from initial Glasgow Outcome Scale, 49% of moderately injured had moderate disabilities at 3 months, and 10% severe. In the mildly injured patients, 78% made good recoveries, 22% were left with moderate disabilities, and none with severe.

Dikmen et al., (1986) evaluated 20 consecutive patients with minor head injury compared to an uninjured control group at 1 and 12 months, on neuropsychological, psychological and adaptive functioning measures. The authors found that minor head injured patients express a multitude of behavioral difficulties, which improve significantly over time, and are attributable to other factors in addition to the head injury. Other system injuries contributed to disabilities in everyday life, including return to work. The authors also noted that other studies with different findings did not control as stringently for prior head injuries. One criticism of this study, which the authors acknowledge is also a problem in the literature, is that the psychosocial/adaptive living indices were largely subjective. A second criticism is that the entire sample size was small, and the one patient who dropped out and was unavailable for 1 year follow-up could have significantly contributed to results.

Bornstein (1989) studied the relationships among severity of injury, neuropsychological deficits, and emotional disturbances in 124 patients with traumatic brain injury sustained in work-related accidents. Sixty-four percent met criteria for mild head injuries. The study found a significant relationship between the degree of neuropsychological deficits, measured by a traditional assessment battery (Halsted-Reitan) and emotional/behavioral deficits, measured by MMPI scores. Impairment in the neuropsychological battery was significantly related to several MMPI scales including the hysteria, depression, hypochondrias, psychosthemia, and schizophrenia scales. The duration of interval between injury and examination was not significantly related to either neuropsychological or emotional indices. There was also no association between degree of neuropsychological deficit and any of a number of neurological injury-related variables, such as duration of retrograde and post-traumatic amnesia, and duration of unconsciousness.

Bernstein et al., also pointed out that, since compensation was not a factor in this study, the relationships of neuropsychological and emotional disturbances supported other reports in the literature suggesting that compensation is not necessarily a factor in these cases (McKinlay et al., 1983).

Because mild brain injury symptoms are so subjective, accurate diagnosis and evaluation of outcome or "recovery" is often more controversial when there are financial gains available to individuals presenting with symptoms. Jones et al., (1992) attempted to mitigate patient subjectivity by relying on surveys of primary care physicians providing continuing medical care to post-mild head injury patients. They surveyed 122 physicians who cared for 256 patients presenting with symptoms of mild head injury in emergency rooms of two community hospitals in Michigan. Of these, 192 (75%) were judged to have experienced mild traumatic brain injuries. Of the total physicians surveyed, 55% responded, and indicated that 21% of those patients were experiencing post-traumatic brain injury symptoms from 2 to 6 months after injury. These data match others reported in the literature.

Hugenholtz et al., (1988) synopsized findings on recovery of cognitive functions, and conducted one of the best controlled studies of function in mild head injury. They measured recovery of simple and complex reaction time in controls and patients with mild head injury. Their data support those generally found in the literature with some differences. They found no significant initial impairments of slowed information processing (measured by simple reaction time) but significant impairments of attention (measured by a choice reaction time test) for subjects with mild head injuries. Symptoms typically described in the literature, recovered over 3 months, whereas deficits in attention persisted. As with many other studies, this study did not attempt a finer analysis of cognitive/behavioral deficits as affected by type of neuropathology or injury. Despite the limitations, on outcome studies such as those reviewed, as noted in prior sections in practice there are three major subpopulations of mild head injuries:

1. Individuals experiencing a mild brain injury with some or many of the sequela as listed in Table 6.2, who experience symptoms for anywhere from hours to 3 months post-injury and then recover to "normal" pre-injury functioning. This group represents the vast majority of mild head injuries with associated brain injuries, estimated at 75-90%.
2. A very small proportion, estimated at 1-3% of those initially presenting with mild head injuries who experience severe deterioration due to a variety of pathologies (slow intracranial bleed, increased intracerebral pressure due to ventricular damage or brain stem swelling, etc.) which may produce coma and death, if untreated.
3. A modest size population, estimated as high as 20%, but difficult to accurately estimate, who have significant "mild" brain injury sequela lasting months, years, or a lifetime. This population actually reflects an array of disabilities with varying levels and types of sequelae based on the diverse pathologies possible in mild head injury. Some undefined percentage of these patients experience significant disruptions/disturbances in their lives due to adverse social, emotional, or employment action which occur during their relatively brief period of recovery. Such cases are particularly challenging to the medilegal expert, as signs/diagnostics of brain injury may have disappeared but residual effects of psychosocial and emotional/behavioral functions endure.

From practice or medi-legal viewpoints, most patients in category 1 above, recover with little adverse impact on their daily lives.

Patients in category 2, who severely deteriorate, are usually reclassified as having moderate or severe brain injuries, with clearly identified pathologies and treatment needs.

The problem population is category 3 above, who present challenges in diagnosing and treating sequelae which may or may not be caused by neurological, or psychological/psychiatric, or other physiological factors, and/or which may be greatly impacted by the individual's physical and social/emotional environments, including the possibilities for secondary gain.

Diagnostics

The array of diagnostic technology which may be used in mild head injuries is the same as that used in all neurologic disorders, including moderate and severe head injuries. However, in mild head injuries, diagnoses are more difficult, and diagnostic procedures are often not utilized, because the initial case presentation in the emergency room is judged not to warrant them, or the patient returns at a later date and presents to a part of the health care system, (psychiatry, psychology) which is not alerted to consider head injuries as a primary disorder.

Table 6.4 lists diagnostic techniques available for use in mild head injury. After reviewing issues of specific diagnostics in detail, general concerns and recommendations for differential diagnosis will be summarized.

Despite the continuous improvements in diagnostic techniques for neurologic disorders over the past decade, significant problems in accurate diagnoses in mild head injuries persist. Before reviewing specific techniques, some general issues warrant discussion.

TABLE 6.4 *Diagnostic Technologies for Mild Brain Injury*

Emergency room/trauma screening	• Severe vs mild head injury
Screening for pre-injury pathologies, problems	• Interviews - patient, significant others • Records review
Neurologic examinations	• Executive functioning screening • Attention and memory screening
Neuroimaging	• Computerized tomography • Magnetic resonance imaging • Position emission tomography • Single photon emission computerized tomography
Physiatric examinations	• Extracranial vascular, neural • Skeletomuscular examinations
Sensory evaluations	• Labyrinthine • Vision • Hearing • Olfactory screening
EEGS and evoked potentials	• Gross cortical dysfunction • Sensory dysfunctions • Subcortical (brainstem) • Attentional deficits
Neuropsychological evaluations	• Executive functions • Memory • Information processing speed
Neurobehavioral	• Situational assessments • Post traumatic stress disorder • Collateral (family) assessments

The first general problem concerns accurate and timely diagnosis of a "mild" head injury which deteriorates into a more severe injury due to a developing pathology, such as an intracranial bleed or increased intracerebral pressure. Issues in these cases are discussed elsewhere in this text, as they involve misdiagnosis of moderate to severe traumatic brain injury. Two points are worth noting herein. One is that continuous and informed monitoring of neurobehavioral signs and symptoms is the best safeguard in these cases. A second issue is that the diagnostic utility of even very specific and accurate procedures, such as CT scans and neuropsychological exams depends upon the timing of their use.

In practice, there are enormous variations in decisions regarding timing of diagnostics. For example, a neuropsychological evaluation conducted within a few days of a mild head injury may show executive and/or memory deficits which will largely or completely resolve over 30-90 days. Likewise, a CT scan done immediately after injury may miss a very slow intracranial bleed developing over days or weeks. The author has experience with traumatic cases in which executive, memory, and emotional/behavioral symptoms developed over a period of weeks after a mild head injury. In one such case, the patient presented to a psychiatric facility two months after a temporal blow in a car accident, and was not accurately diagnosed until a CT scan two years later revealed a large unilateral fronto-temporal hematoma. This would probably not have been detected by an initial CT scan, but would have if the CT scan had been done after symptoms had developed over a one to two month period.

Emergency Room Screening

Emergency room staff are typically well trained in triage and prioritization, and are focused on diagnosing severe traumatic brain injuries, and those injuries which initially present as mild, but may deteriorate rapidly or gradually into severe and life-threatening conditions.

Typical ER evaluations of post concussion or mild head injury patients include a neurological exam which determines the patient's overall state of consciousness and the integrity of sensory, motor, and basic cognitive functions (Tyson, 1986). Depending upon the institution's practices and/or the screening physician's judgment, more extensive evaluations may or may not occur. A very small percentage of patients who fit the classic definition of mild head injury are admitted, and all but an even smaller percent are released after 1-3 days of observation.

However, growing awareness of problems of misdiagnosis have led some institutions to adopt more sensitive and extensive screenings for mild traumatic brain injuries which require additional diagnostics as indicated in this review.

In addition to medical staff evaluations, the nature and extent of initial information and training provided to patients and families has significant implications for mild head injury.

It has been the author's experience with many prominent hospitals that emergency room screening and follow-up instruction to families addresses only signs of severe brain injury. Handouts or instructions on what to observe or what to do about mild TBI are often not used. This phenomenon is understandable, since MTBI does not merit the attention of severe life-threatening injuries. Moreover, the most critical concern of ER medical staff is that patients and families be informed of signs of deterioration due to severe sequelae.

However, enlightened ER staff are beginning to utilize revised instructions to families in order to alert families to the potential sequelae of MTBI and to suggest strategies ranging from tips the family and victim can use to reduce discomfort and problems to red flags which require medical or rehabilitation treatment.

Table 6.5 compares an ER handout designed for severe TBI recently received from a major teaching hospital in the Northeast with a handout adapted by the author and subsequently adopted at the same hospital, designed to screen for mild TBI. The first handout is typical of ER instruction packets. In contrast, the mild TBI screening provides an ER handout which has been developed for use at another hospital, which addresses potential sequelae and

TABLE 6.5 *Part A: Instructions to Patients and Families Concerning Head Injuries*

Although the patient has been thoroughly examined for evidence of head injury, there are certain signs of trouble which may appear in the next 48 hours. The examining physician considers it safe to allow the patient to return home. However, please observe him/her carefully during the next 48 hours, and telephone us should any of the following signs of trouble develop. Before leaving the hospital, be sure that you have had all of the signs of trouble listed below explained to you by the examining physician and that all of your questions have been answered.

SIGNS OF TROUBLE

1. Excessive Drowsiness: The patient may well be exhausted by the ordeal surrounding the injury, but should be easily aroused by methods that you would ordinarily employ to awaken him from a deep sleep. If you cannot do this, please notify the doctor.

2. Persistent Vomiting: Persons will, in many cases, vomit one or more times following a severe head injury. Should the vomiting recur more than once or twice, or should it begin again hours after it has ceased, notify the doctor.

3. Pupil Inequality: If one pupil appears to be larger than the other, notify the doctor.

Normal Not Normal

4. Unsteadiness: If the patient does not use either arm or leg as well as previously, or is unsteady in walking, notify the doctor.

5. Slurred Speech: Should speech become slurred or the patient is apparently unable to talk, notify the doctor.

6. Severe Headache: If a severe headache occurs, particularly if it increases in severity and is not relieved by aspirin or Tylenol, notify the doctor.

7. Double Vision: Should he/she complain of "seeing double" or should you detect any failure of the eyes to move together appropriately, notify the doctor.

Continued

8. Convulsions: Should a convulsion occur, place the patient on one side and where he cannot fall. Be sure there is ample room for him to breathe. Stay with the patient until the convulsion begins to subside, and notify the doctor as soon as possible and return to the Emergency Department.

9. If the patient seems to recover and worsens, notify the doctor.

On the night following the head injury, or during any nap, it may be advisable to awaken the patient every four hours and look for any of those danger signs. Your doctor will tell you if this is necessary.

Please call or return to the Emergency Department if you have any questions or problems arise.

TABLE 6.5 *Part B: Mild Head Injury*

More Signs to Watch for:

You have received the handout on SIGNS OF TROUBLE which may appear within the next 48 hours, and which indicate you may have a severe problem and should immediately contact your Doctor or the Emergency Room. There are also signs which indicate that you should consider a reevaluation by your doctor or this hospital, because you may have a "MILD" or minor head injury. That is, these signs may indicate minor trauma to brain or nerve cells (not that "you are going crazy"). Sometimes minor head trauma can produce significant problems if not treated. Here are some things to watch for, especially if they are marked changes since the injury. If they last longer than two or three weeks, and are interfering in your daily home life or work, you should consider a reevaluation:

Signs:

Headaches
Dizziness
Ringing in the ear(s)
Fatigue
Problems in: concentration, memory, organizing activities or things
Problems reading
Problems learning new things, skills, directions, routines
Problems finding the right words, expressing yourself

Continued

Reduced ability to think; slowed thinking; confusion
Reduced insight
Irritability, depression, anxiety
Increased emotionality (laugh, cry more easily; large or fast mood swings)
Saying/doing things others take offense at

Self or Family Observation:

"You are not the same person"
"Your judgment is off"
"You are missing things, reactions, in conversations"
"You can't seem to accomplish anything", "Spinning wheels"
"Every little thing takes effort"

Again, these MAY indicate that you have persisting symptoms of mild brain injury. If you are interested in a reevaluation, contact:

---

suggested responses specific for MTBI. This handout was developed in part by the author and other colleagues, based on the NHIF pamphlet, "The Unseen Injury, Minor Head Trauma: An Introduction for Patients and Families" (Kay, 1986), with added materials from a number of sources, including the author's personal experiences. The NHIF pamphlet alone represents an excellent guide, and is recommended as an addition to be given to families. The handout in Table 6.5 is suggested because it presents an eye-catching format similar to the typical ER screen for severe TBI, and may prompt families to use the NHIF pamphlet or seek professional advice.

Screening for Pre-Injury Problems

Symptoms reported by a patient which are ascribed to a recent mild head injury may be the result of any one or a combination of several prior medical or psychological problems. The practitioner seeking to provide differential diagnosis must thoroughly evaluate prior history and potential contributors to the presenting symptoms.

In addition to a thorough review of prior medical histories, review of prior work histories, school records, military records, and social histories may be useful. The practitioner should be reviewing these histories for indicators of pre-existing psychological problems, including neuropsychological problems such as Attention Deficit Disorder, with or without hyperactivity, traditional psychiatric or psychological problems which may produce symptoms similar to those in mild head injury. Psychosomatic profiles are especially important to identify, and the notation of the number and severity of life stressors, for example, as part of a standard psychological DSM-III evaluation, can be useful. Potential substance abuse may also require review, which can be detected by traditional professional evaluations combined with drug screening.

Prior head injuries must also be carefully sought and evaluated in constructing histories. Patients and families may not have recognized a prior injury as severe if the patient wasn't subjected to hospitalization and/or intense treatment. Asking questions carefully, for example, "have you ever gone to the emergency room for a blow to the head", or "were you ever knocked unconscious or dizzy" may reveal prior incidents when the question "have you ever been diagnosed or treated for a head injury" will not.

Prior injuries do not rule out the possibility that a recent incident has produced significant additional pathology and symptoms. In fact, the literature suggests that: 1) individuals with head injuries have a higher risk of having subsequent injuries, and 2) the results of subsequent injuries are often more severe, as injuries have cumulative impacts, and the "cerebral reserve" is diminished (Ewing et al., 1980).

Neurologic examinations typically evaluate gross states of consciousness, and many specific sensory, motor, reflexive, perceptual and cognitive functions, for signs of peripheral and/or central nervous system dysfunction (Cooper, 1993). The accuracy of diagnosing traumatic brain injury at initial presentation is a function of the severity of injury, and the sensitivity of the exam. Whereas severe injury and corresponding sequelae are more readily identified and detailed, symptoms of mild head injuries may not be easily revealed unless the medical examiner utilizes procedures designed to detect disorders of cognition, attention, memory, and executive functions. The typical initial indicators of "post concussion syndrome" in the emergency room, including slowed information processing and/or motor responses are also detectable in neurologic exams, although these typically resolve in a manner of hours or days, leaving the less easily detected symptoms of executive, memory, or attention functions noted above.

Neuroimaging

The utility and limitations of CT scans for a spectrum of head injuries has been discussed by many authors.

Marshal et al., (1992) provided one of the largest and best controlled studies of patients under the auspices of the National Traumatic Coma Data Bank. Their overall findings confirm the utility of CT scans in managing cases, and the relationship of the volume status of the brain to predicted outcomes. The importance of obtaining serial vs. "snapshot" CT scans at initial admission and the utility of MRI's is also reviewed.

As prominent authors, such as Teasdale (1992) have pointed out, the match between imaging and pathology is incomplete, and rests, for an individual patient, on assumed relationships versus established facts. However, for more severe head injuries, more defined CT analysis combined with other key indicators, such as intracerebral pressure, are increasingly better predictors for long term outcomes. In mild head injuries CT will continue into the foreseeable future in a prominent and commonly used diagnostic role of identifying mass lesions for surgical intervention before severe sequelae develop.

Dacey et al., (1986) conducted a prospective study of 610 patients who fit the generally accepted definition of mild head injury, with transient post-trauma loss of consciousness, and GCS of 13 to 15. They found that 3% of these patients deteriorated to the point where they required neurosurgical treatment. These data match well with other large scale studies of patients who present with "minor" or "mild" head injuries, and who deteriorate.

The Dacey et al., study (1986) provides data supporting the use of skull x-rays and CT scans in managing "mild"head injuries. One factor is that 3% of the patients with GCS of 13 to 15 required surgical interventions. A second is that an abnormal skull x-ray increased by a factor of 20 the probability that a patient required neurosurgery. However, 20% of the patients who developed intracranial hematomas had normal skull radiographs.

Finally, Dacey et al., provide a welcome review of cost-effectiveness of alternative management schemes, which argues for use of CT scans or skull films to determine which patients should be admitted for observation. They also point out the limitation of all current management schemes. One example of an unusual case was a patient who deteriorated over a 30-day period as the result of subarachnoid cyst which apparently was asymptomatic until damaged by the minor head injury.

Jeret et al., (1993) have recently published an extensive prospective study of 712 consecutive patients seen in a New York emergency room, to assess the relationship of CT scans with other clinical predictors of "mild" head injury. Patients were seen within 24 hours of injury, with well defined loss of consciousness (LOC) and Glasgow Coma Scale of 15. CT scans found lesions in 67, or 9.4%, of which 32 patients had multiple lesions. Two required neurosurgical interventions, and one expired. CT findings correlated positively with older ages, Caucasian race, basilar skull fracture, and auto-pedestrian accidents, but did not correlate with other variables, including length of amnesia (retro- or anterograde), digit spans (forward or reverse, as short term memory measures), neurologic examinations, or subjective complaints. Jeret et al., (1993) also noted that in the three most severe cases, CT scans were not instrumental in indicating surgeries, as other clinical symptoms clearly signalled the need for surgical interventions.

Comparisons of CT and MRI with SPECT have clearly indicated SPECT to be more sensitive in detecting small and functional lesions. For example, Goldenberg et al., (1992), correlated SPECT scans with neuropsychological evaluations on thirty-six patients with severe head injuries. SPECT scans conducted from 7 to 66 months post injury detected lower flow indices in patients bilaterally in orbitofrontal and anterograde regions, but higher flow values in others. Thalamic flows were lower, but not significantly so. Tests of secondary memory did not correlate well with any flow values. Temporal lobe flows correlated only with vocabulary test scores. Executive function tests correlated with frontal cortical flows, but stronger relations were found with thalamic values. Expected correlations between memory tests and hippocampal flow rates may have been masked by variations in hippocampal flow due to spontaneous mental activities during SPECT.

Comparisons of the sensitivity of SPECT, CT and MRI technology in detecting lesions have been increasingly clear regarding the relative merits and shortfalls of each. An example is the recent study by Newton et al., (1992) which compared the three techniques in 19 patients with severe head injury 3 to 36 months post injury. SPECT detected 43 perfusion deficits, MRI 21 focal lesions, and CT 13. Of the 43 SPECT lesions, 31 were not detected on either CT or MRI. Five of 21 MRI detected lesions were unique to MRI's, and CT detected only 4 lesions not otherwise found. The number of SPECT defects and the global cerebral flood flow correlated with functional status of the patient, measured by the Glasgow Outcome Scale, extended version. The authors note the relative merits of SPECT in detecting smaller functional lesions, whereas CT is still both widely available and invaluable in early acute-stage detection of neuropathological processes such as hematomas and hydrocephalus which require surgical intervention.

Levin et al., (1987), studying 20 patients with minor or moderate head injuries, evaluated the relative sensitivities of MRI and CT as correlated with neurobehavioral sequelae. MRI scans demonstrated 44 more intracranial lesions than did CT scans in 17 patients, and estimated greater lesion volumes than CT scans in most. Nine (9) of these cases had more MRI lesions than found on CT, and 3 cases had neither MRI nor CT findings of lesions. Neuropsychological assessments at 24 hours post MRI (unless confusion or PTA prohibited) included tests specifically designed for frontal and temporal lobe functions: concept formation and problem solving flexibility (modified card-sorting), verbal fluency, design fluency, verbal selective reminding for long term memory, and a spatial (non-verbal) analog for long term non-verbal memory. Initial MRI's were related to neuropsychological assessments during hospitalizations. Significant reductions in MRI lesion sizes and neuropsychological improvements were found for the 13 patients who returned at 1 month for follow-up. Decreasing numbers of cases at 3 months make interpretation of further findings difficult. However, 2 of the 13 patients followed at 3 months had not returned to work.

Among other findings, the authors noted that MRI technology improvements may allow detection of additional or larger lesions, or more persisting lesions, than those available. They also noted that MRI was not helpful in disclosing lesions requiring surgical evacuation.

Levin et al., (1992) subsequently evaluated the utility of CT and MRI scans in 50 cases of mild (40) and moderate (10) brain injury followed for 3 months post injury. Mild was defined as GCS of 13-15, loss of consciousness of 20 minutes or less and no deterioration. Moderate was defined as admission or lowest GCS 9-12 with no deterioration. In addition to a CT scan during admission, MRI's and neurobehavioral assessments measuring a number of cognitive and behavioral functions were measured at admission, and one and three months post injury. Neurobehavioral tests focused on executive and memory functions.

Of the total, 4 cases (80%) had intracranial abnormalities in initial MRI's; 13 of these had normal CT's, and 26 (52%) had MRI's showing more lesions than CT. One patient had identical CT and MRI findings. Nine patients had CT lesions not seen on MRI. Ten patients (20%) had normal images on CT and MRI.

Parenchymal lesions found on MRI were primarily fronto-temporal. However, the size of parenchymal lesion was unrelated to severity of impaired consciousness. Individual patients with resolved front-temporal lesions tended to have a higher proportion of tests with affective scores than patients who had no initial MRI lesions. The authors also noted a tendency for patients to move over time from pervasive to specific symptoms. These findings were limited by a small number of cases studied, which was complicated by a failure to return for reassessment by a significant number of patients.

A proliferation of neuroimaging studies is providing increasing evidence on the relationships among detectable indicators of abnormal structure and physiology. At this time, the primary value to practitioners is in detecting those conditions which need intervention, such as developing hematomas, masses, or pressure-induced displacements of brain tissue. The value of neuroimaging in prescribing treatment or predicting outcomes in mild head injury awaits substantially more development of literature.

Other Screenings

As Zasler (1992) has described in detail, physiatric evaluation in order to distinguish extracranial vs. intracranial sources of symptoms, particularly pain and sensory-motor dysfunctions may be critical for accurate diagnoses. Particular concerns for the practitioner or medi-legal evaluator are referred pain, such as occipital neuralgia, which may masquerade as "intracranial" or migraine headache, myofascial pain disorders, labyrinthine (particularly in temporal injuries), and peripheral nerve disorders, all of which may present as symptoms of brain injury, but which have extracranial pathologies requiring very specific treatment approaches.

In addition to screening for vision and hearing, which are often components of neurologic or physiatric exams, screenings for dysfunctions of smell and taste can sometimes confirm a brain injury. The relationship of anosmia to ortibito-frontal damage and potential predictive value of anosmia has been well reviewed by Varney and Menafee (1993). There appears to be growing evidence that patients with anosmia have more significant deficits, characterized by poorer long-term outcomes, compared to patients without anosmia.

Electroencephalogram

Electrocephalographic (EEG) and evoked potentials, which are averaged EEG responses to specific stimuli, have received less attention in the literature and in practice, as neuroimaging techniques have become more accessible and precise. There are, however, clear and significant changes in EEG with temporary and permanent brain injury, which parallel changes in neurobehavioral and neuroimaging indicators of dysfunction. The EEG changes may reflect gross widespread or relatively focal changes in cortical function. Evoked potentials reflect changes in specific sensory pathways, including visual, auditory, and somasensory systems. Brain stem auditory evoked responses (recorded from scalp electrodes, but detecting electrical responses in brain stem auditory centers) are useful in indicating brain stem functional status. Evoked responses can also be utilized to detect dysfunctions of attention, which are reflected by alterations in selected components of the evoked potential (P300) (Heinze et al., 1992; Livinger et al., 1990; Levin & Eisenberg, 1988).

Neuropsychological Evaluations

Thorough neuropsychological associations which assess for deficits in those cognitive and neurobehavioral areas found to be affected by mild brain injuries are by far the most useful diagnostic procedures for detailing symptoms and problems. While there are not standardized assessments which are universally accepted for use in mild head injury cases, there is a growing literature and growing practice of using tests or subtests of larger "batteries" which focus on commonly diagnosed problems of memory, attention, and executive functions. For example, tests such as Rey's Complex Figure Test, with Osterreith's Analysis (sometimes referred to as the Rey-Osterreith Test), the Verbal Fluency Test, and the Wisconsin Card Sorting Test, among others, are particularly sensitive to executive dysfunctions (Lezak, 1993).

For practicing professionals who are "consumers" of neuropsychological evaluations, several key concerns should be addressed whenever neuropsychological testing is conducted and interpreted. The first is that, unless tests or subtests which specifically and sensitively assess for executive, attentional, and memory functions are given, deficits may be missed. It is not uncommon to review records of cases in which psychological evaluations which included a "neuropsychological screening" did not find symptoms of injury, which were later definitely revealed by more sensitive tests.

Executive functions are difficult to diagnose, as most testing situations attempt to structure, organize, and motivate the subject to perform in the tests (Lezak, 1987). These organizational functions may be those specific areas which are deficient, and so the test may remove the opportunity for the deficit to appear. Newly created tests such as the "Tinkertoy Test" (Bayless et al., 1989) are specifically designed to detect such dysfunctions.

A second issue concerns a diverse set of behaviors which involve executive functions in the "psychosocial" arena. Varney and Menefee (1993) have provided a detailed overview of these disorders and the difficulties in diagnosing and treating them. The behaviors in question are difficult to measure but critically important to success in everyday life, including empathy, judgment, impulse control, social appropriateness, and others. The executive functions which monitor and regulate motivational, emotional and social repertoires, are difficult to assess in testing, as formal evaluations are not designed to assess such deficits, especially if they are limited in scope or severity. "Situational Assessments", described below, are much more sensitive to psychosocial deficits (Jacobs & Hart, 1993).

A third issue concerns the separation of neurological from psychiatric and/or environmental contributors to presenting symptoms. Whereas it is widely accepted in the literature and practice that all three sets of variables may interact to produce severe problems, there are no easily accessible or generally accepted methods or protocols to separate their relative contributions. Careful histories for pre-injury problems, as noted above, may assist in identifying review of prior psychiatric/psychological contributors.

Assessing the relative impacts of psychosocial environmental factors is largely left to the skill of the evaluator.

Overall, of all the diagnostic techniques used in mild head injury, neuropsychological assessments which assess potential executive, attention, memory, and psychosocial functions offer the most sensitive, reliable, and specific information on deficits.

Situational Assessments

The limitations of neuropsychological, neurological, physiatric, psychiatric, and other evaluations in detecting executive and psychosocial deficits, and in separating out relative contributions of neurologic vs. environmental factors, have lead researchers and practitioners to utilize techniques termed "situational assessments" (Hart & Jacobs, 1993; Burke et al., 1991). Patients are placed in real world or analog situations of daily living, work, or social activities, and their behavior is carefully observed and recorded. Typically, such assessments utilize particular events, people, or environmental conditions designed to assess suspected deficits uncovered in interviews or formal evaluations. This approach produces reliable data without the structure of formal testing which may mask executive or psychosocial deficits. Evaluations may be conducted in the patient's home, at the workplace, or during a brief residential inpatient admission.

The advantages of situational assessments are many. One is the evaluator's ability to detect deficits due to task demands which require executive functions of planning and implementing activities and related attentional and memory capabilities, all necessary to live normally and work productively. A second advantage is that social stressors which are also usually controlled for in medical and psychological evaluations can be assessed for impact on cognitive and emotional/social behavior. A third is that environmental variables can be assessed. For example, the impact of noise and multiple social demands in the workplace, which may adversely impact performance but again are usually controlled for and so absent in typical exams, can be evaluated. A fourth is that any fluctuations in cognitive and psychosocial functioning over the course of the day/night can be assessed. Subtle but significant problems in emotional behavior or cognition, in regulatory functions such as eating and sleeping, which have not been reported, may appear in situational assessments. Finally, situational assessments may be extremely useful in evaluating potential compensatory or skill-building techniques which are critical for rehabilitation (Burke, et al., 1991).

Whiplash

The phenomenon of "whiplash", a relatively common complaint of individuals struck from the rear in automobile accidents, deserves special comment.

A small, difficult to define percentage of common whiplash patients develop severe debilitation. Yarnell and Rossie (1988) studied 27 such whiplash patients who were at least 1 year post injury, and who otherwise had no physical or neuropsychological sequelae of an auto accident. These patients would not have been categorized as "mild" head injuries, as there were none reporting loss of consciousness or anything more than a brief period of being "dazed" at the time of injury. CT scans, MRI's, EEG's, brain stem auditory evoked responses all failed to detect significant indicators of neurologic injury, with one or two exceptions in each type of evaluation. A large and comprehensive neuropsychological testing battery (the Halstead Reitan Battery with additions) was administered, and found that 68% of the patients were neurologically impaired. All patients had previously been employed, but one year post injury had significant changes in employment status, with 50% not working and the other 50% working at reduced levels of hours or income. Of 14 patients who completed the Minnesota Multiphasic Personality Inventory, 8 profiles were abnormal on the Goldberg index (a weighted score based on depression), anxiety and character disturbance. The authors ranked neuropsychological tests by sensitivity. They also noted that no correlations were found between return to work and sex, age, length of time since accident, Halstead Impairment index, or active involvement in a lawsuit.

A percentage of "whiplash" victims may be viewed as a subset of the mild head injury population who have experienced either diffuse axonal injury or cerebral (frontal or temporal, usually) contusions. Issues of identifying and treating extracranial (ligament, vascular, neural) vs. brain injuries are the same as those for any mild head injury, as discussed throughout the chapter. Psychiatric evaluation for the identification of serious problems such as vetebrobasilar insufficiency or anterior or posterior sympathetic plexus tearing may be critical for appropriate treatment.

Treatment

Many prominent clinicians and researchers have provided overviews of rehabilitation and treatment of mild head injuries (Boake et al., 1991, Levin & Eisenberg, 1988, Cooper, 1993). All strongly have indicated that educating patients and families about the causes, symptoms, and management techniques is critical to successful rehabilitation. Without such education, patients and families may react inappropriately to emerging symptoms, resulting in exacerbated stressors, inappropriate treatments, and poorer outcomes (Davidoff et al., 1988). Some authors have recommended that patients take a period of leave from work for two weeks and reduce overall schedule and activity loads, to avoid stresses and facilitate recovery (Levin & Eisenberg, 1988). Newly developing treatment programs for mild head injury patients emphasize anxiety reduction and education in assisting patients to resume normal family and work activities (Sporadeo, 1994).

For specific pain, sensory, motor, cognitive, or behavioral dysfunctions, targeted rehabilitation treatments are prescribed. Several authors have reviewed treatment approaches for executive, memory, and psychosocial dysfunctions (Burke et al., 1991; Freeman et al., 1992; Goodwin & Bolton, 1991 Hart & Jacobs, 1993; Kreutzer & Wehman, 1991; Sholberg et al., 1993). In general, the emerging literature indicates that a variety of compensatory devices and strategies and skill-teaching approaches may be successful in remediating sequelae of mild head injuries.

For the medilegal practitioner, selecting among or evaluating the success of rehabilitation programs should focus on practical, functional, and clearly specified objectives. For example, a program with a stated objective of improving memory or cognitive retraining would not meet these criteria. A program would meet such criteria if it proposed a stated objective of returning a client to work in a specified job for x hours per week with a defined level of support or an objective of reducing the amount of a client's needed supervision or improving a client's performance on routine tasks such as carrying out shopping trips, household activities, etc. Programs designed to meet clear functional objectives should start by evaluating the client's strengths and deficits, and the performance needs and potential problems in the discharge environments. Treatment or training should be clearly designed to address needs in the discharge environments. For example, a proper approach would not have a client practicing memory exercises or cognitive retraining at a computer station, but might have a client learning to use a day planner (much more explicit and frequently used than those the author and reader might use) and other memory-aides (checklists, computer prompted steps of key tasks, etc.) to function at home or in the work place.

Two other key criteria include objective measurement of progress along the way, with data used to adjust treatments, and development of useful, non-burdensome, but often needed supports in the home and work place (or school). Functional, discharge-driven approaches have been well discussed in detail by other authors (Burke et al., 1991; Hart & Jacobs, 1993).

The overall approach to treatment of mild head injuries should assist patients and families in understanding that, although focal and/or mild behavioral sequelae may be permanent, proper supports and use of compensatory strategies and skills will make the sequelae manageable, with minimal impact on quality of life.

Summary

The term mild head injury actually refers to multiple disorders which produce a diverse array of physical, neurological, and behavioral sequelae. This chapter reviewed issues and practices in the definitions, diagnoses, and outcomes, and treatment of mild head injuries.

Until this disorder benefits from substantial development of new diagnostic technologies, the medilegal practitioner is advised to approach each case of mild head injury with great caution.

References

Adams, J.H., Graham, D.I., Murray, L.S. et al, (1982). Diffuse axonal injury due to non-missle head injury in humans: An analysis of 45 cases. *Annals of Neurology,* 12, 557-563.

Barlow, C.F. (1984). Headaches and migraine in childhood. *Clinics in Developmental Medicine*, 91, 6-11.

Barth, J., Macciocchi, S. & Giordanni, B.(1983). Neuropsychological sequelae of minor head injury. *Neurosurgery,* 13, 529-533.

Bayless, J., Varney, N. & Roberts, R. (1989). Tinker Toy Test performance and vocational outcome in patients with closed head injuries. *Journal of Clinical and Experimental Neuropsycology*, 11, 913-917

Bennett, T. (1988). Post-traumatic headaches: Subtypes and behavioral treatments. *Cognitive Rehabilitation*, 6, 34-39.

Blumberg, P.C., Jones, N.R. & North, J.B. (1989). Diffuse axonal injury in head trauma. *Journal of Neurology, Neurosurgury and Psychiatry*, 52, 838-841.

Boake, C., Bobetic, K.M., Bontke, C.F. (1991). Rehabilitation of the patient with mild traumatic brain injury. *Neurorehabilitation*, 1, 70-78.

Bornstein, R.N., Miller, H.B. and Van Schoar, J.T. (1989). Neuropsychological deficit and emotional disturbance in head injured patients. *Journal of Neurosurgery*, 70, 509-513.

Burke, W.H., Zencius, A., Wesolowski, M.D. & Doubleday, F. (1991). Improving executive function disorders in brain-injured clients. *Brain Injury,* 5, 241-252.

Colohan, A.R. & Oyesiku, N.M. (1992). Moderate head injury: An overview. *Journal of Neurotrauma*, 9, 5259-5264.

Cooper, P. (Editor) (1993). *Head Injury (Third Edition).* Baltimore, MD: Williams & Wilkins.

Dacey, R.G., Alves, W.M., Rimel, R.W., Winn, H.R. & Jane, J.A. (1986). Neurosurgical complications after apparently minor head injury. *Journal of Neurosurgery*, 65, 203-210.

Davidoff, D.A., Kessler, H.R., Laibstain, D.F., & Mark, V.H. (1988). Neurobehavioral sequelae of minor head injury: A consideration of post-concussive syndrome versus post-traumatic stress disorder. *Cognitive Rehabilitation,* March-April, 8-13.

Dikmen, S., Machamer, J. & Temkin, N. (1993). Psychosocial outcome in patients with moderate to severe head injury: Two-year follow-up. *Brain Injury,* 7, 113-124.

Dickmen, S., McLean, A. & Temkin, N. (1986). Neuropsychological and psychosocial consequences of minor head injury. *Journal of Neurology, Neurosurgery and Psychiatry*, 49, 1227-1232.

Ewing, R., McCarthy, D., Gronwall D. & Wrightson, P. (1980). Persisting effects of minor head injury observable during hypoxic stress. *Journal of Clinical Neuropsychology*, 2, 147-155.

Fisher, J. (1985). Cognitive and behavioral consequences of closed head injury. *Seminars in Neurology,* 5, 1-8.

Freeman, M.R., Mittenberg, W., Dicownden, M. & Bat-Ami, M. (1992). Executive and compensatory memory retraining in traumatic brain injury. *Brain Injury,* 6, 65-70.

Genarelli, T.A., Spielman, G.M., Langfitt, J.W. et al, (1982a). Influence of the type of intracranial lesion on outcome for severe head injury: A multicenter study using a new classification system. *Journal of Neurosurgery,* 56, 26-32.

Genarelli, T.A., Thibault, L.E., Adams, J.H. et al, (1982b). Diffuse axonal injury and traumatic coma in the primate. *American Neurology*, 12, 564-574.

Haas, D. & Lourie, H. (1988). Trauma triggered migraine: An explanation for common neurological attacks after mild head injury. *Journal of Neurosurgery*, 68, 181-188.

Hart, T. & Jacobs, H.E. (1993). Rehabilitation and management of behavioral disturbances following frontal lobe injury. *Journal of Head Trauma Rehabilitation*, 8, 1-12.

Heinze, H.J., Munte, T.F., Gobiet, et al, (1992). Parallel and serial visual search after closed head injury: Electrophysiological evidence for perceptual dysfunctions. *Neuropsychologia,* 30, 495-514.

Hugenholtz, H., Stuss, D.T., Stethem, L.L. & Richard, M.T. (1988). How long does it take to recover from mild concussion. *Neurosurgery*, 22, 853-858.

Jeret, J., Mandell, M., Anziska, B., Liritz, M., et al, (1993). Clinical predictors of abnormality disclosed by computed tomography after mild head injury. *Neurosurgery,* 32, 9-16.

Jones, J.H., Viola, S.L., LaBlan, M.M., Schyroll, W. & Krome, R.L. (1992). The incidence of post minor traumatic brain injury syndrome: A retrospect study of treating physicians. *Archives of Physical Medicine and Rehabilitation*, 73, 145-146.

Kay, T.(1986). *Minor Head Injury: An Introduction for Professionals.* Framingham, MA: National Head Injury Foundation.

Klonoff, P.S., Snow, W.G. & Costa L.D. (1986). Quality of life in patients 2 to 4 years after closed head injury. *Neurosurgery,* 19, 735-743.

Levin, H. (1992). Neurobehavioral recovery. *Journal of Neurotrauma,* 9, S359-S373.

Levin, H.S., Amparo, E., Eisenberg, et al, (1987). Magnetic resonance imaging and computerized tomography in relation to the neurobehavioral sequelae of mild and moderate head injuries. *Journal of Neurosurgery,* 66, 706-713.

Levin, H.S., Eisenberg, H.M. (1988). Post concussional syndrome, *Neurotrauma Medical Report*, 2, 1-3.

Levin, H.S., Eisenberg, H.M. & Benton, A.L. (Eds.). (1989). *Mild Head Injury.* New York, NY: Oxford University Press.

Levin, H.S., Eisenberg, H.M., Benton, A.L. (Eds.). (1991). *Frontal Lobe Function and Dysfunction.* New York, NY: Oxford University Press.

Levin, H.S., Williams, D.H., Eisenberg, H.M., et al, (1992). Serial MRI and Neurobehavioral findings after mild to moderate closed head injury. *Journal of Neurology, Neurosurgery and Psychiatry,* 55, 255-262.

Lezak, M. (1983). *Neuropsychological Assessment.* New York, NY: Oxford University Press.

Lezak, M. (1987). The problem of assessing executive functions. *International Journal Psychology*, 17, 281-297.

Lieninger, B.E., Gramling, S.E., Farrell, A.D., et al, (1990). Neuropsychological deficits in symptomatic minor head injury patients after concussion and mild concussion. *Journal of Neurology, Neurosurgery and Psychiatry,* 53, 293-296.

Marshall, L.F., Marshall, S.B., Klauber, M.R., et al, (1992). The diagnosis of head injury requires a classification based on computed axial tomography. *Journal of Neurotrauma*, 9, S287-S292.

McKinlay, W.W., Brooks, D.N., Bond, M.R. (1983). Post concussional symptoms, financial compensation and outcome of severe blunt head injury. *Journal of Neurology, Neurosurgery and Psychiatry*, 46, 1084-1091.

National Head Injury Foundation (1991). *The Unseen Injury - Minor Head Trauma*, Southborough, MA: NHIF.

Povlishock, J.T., Eib, D.E. & Astrue, J. (1992). Axonal response to traumatic brain injury: Reactive axonal change, differentiation and neuroplasticity, *Journal of Neurotrauma,* 9, S189-S200.

Rimel, R.W., Giordani, B., Barth, J.T., et al, (1981). Disability caused by minor head injury. *Neurosurgery,* 9, 221-228.

Rimel, R.W., Giordani, B., Barth, J.T., et al, (1982). Moderate head injury: Completing the spectrum of brain trauma. *Neurosurgery*, 11, 344-351.

Ruff, R.M., Levin, H.S., Marshall, L.F. (1986). Neurobehavioral methods of assessment and the study of outcome in minor head injury. *Journal of Head Trauma Rehabilitation,* 1, 43-52.

Rutherford, W.H. (1989). Post concussion symptoms: Relationship to acute neurologic indices, individual differences, and circumstances of injury. In Levin, H.S., Eisenberg, H.M., Benton, A.L. (Eds.). *Mild Head Injury.* New York, NY: Oxford University Press.

Saigh, P.A. (1992). *Post-traumatic Stress Disorder: A Behavioral Approach to Assessment and Treatment.* DesMoines, IA: Allyn and Bacon.

Saneda, D.L. & Corrigan, J.D. (1992). Predicting clearing of post-traumatic amnesia following closed head injury. *Brain Injury*, 6, 167-174.

Schwab, K., Grafman, J., Salazar, A., Kraft, J. (1993). Residual impairments and work status 15 years after penetrating head injury, *Neurology,* 43, 95-103.

Stuss, D.T. & Benson, D.F. (1986). *The Frontal Lobes.* New York, NY: Rowen Press.

Teasdale, G., Teasdale, E. & Hadley, D. (1992). Computed Tomographic and Magnetic Resonance Imaging classification of head injury. *Journal of Neurotrauma*, 9, S249-S257.

Tyson, G.W. (1988). *Head Injury Management for Providers of Emergency Care.* Baltimore, MD: Williams and Wilkins.

Varney, N.R. & Menefee, L. (1993). Psychosocial and executive deficits following closed head injury: Implications for orbital frontal cortex. *Journal of Head Trauma Rehabilitation*, 8, 32-44.

Varney, N.R. & Menefee, L. (1993). Psychosocial and executive deficits following closed head injury: Implications for orbital frontal cortex. *Journal of Head Trauma Rehabilitation*, 8, 32-44.

Yarnell, P.R. & Rossie, G.V. (1988). Minor whiplash head injury with major debilitation. *Brain Injury*, 2, 255-258.

Zasler, N. & Horne, L. (1992). *Rehabilitation of Post Concussive Disorders.* Philadelphia, PA: Hanley & Belfus.

Bruce L. Bird, Ph.D. - Director of Behavioral Medicine

Dr. Bird is a licensed psychologist and currently the Executive Director of the Institutes for Behavior Resources, a not-for-profit behavioral medicine research center and community-based provider of services for disabled individuals in Baltimore and Washington, D.C. Dr. Bird is on the faculty of the Harvard University School of Medicine. He has published 17 research studies and lectures throughout the U.S. in the areas of behavioral medicine, neurologic case management, community-based treatment and health care reform.

7

PEDIATRIC BRAIN INJURY: ANALYSIS, PLANNING AND MANAGEMENT

Carole Wedel Sellars, Ph.D., CCC
William H. Burke, Ph.D., CRC

Children with brain injuries are complex and challenging cases for forensic rehabilitation specialists. This is true for a variety of reasons which certainly include the reality that hurt children are emotionally explosive. Every adult in the courtroom, hospital and review conference room empathizes with the case by mentally and emotionally holding in their mind as reference their own children, grandchildren, nieces, and nephews. It is always a tragedy of mammoth proportion when a child is hurt. That injury may occur before, during or after birth. At the very least, it negatively influences that child's potential and in moderate and severe cases, it likely will shatter all dreams for a normal life.

The purpose of this chapter is to present information which balances this emotionality with objectivity. In the cases of infants, toddlers and children with brain injuries, a Pediatric Rehabilitation Expert is critical to accurately analyze the child's disabilities and provide thoughtful input into the long term medical, educational, rehabilitative, social-emotional, leisure and vocational needs of the child through his or her lifetime. This role must be assumed by a clinical specialist, a person with continuing clinical opportunity to provide care and follow children with brain injuries long term. In terms of traumatic brain injuries, it is generally society's impression that young adults get brain injuries in motorcycle and car accidents. This chapter's purpose is to remind you that infants, toddlers, preschool children, and teenagers also sustain brain injuries.

Children are verbs. They scoot, crawl, climb, walk, run, jump, skip, ride, play swim, explore, and compete. But children are not childproof. They can't have safety caps put on them. They fall out of windows, off of horses, and into swimming pools; they get hit by cars; they play with guns; they ride in many motorized vehicles; they ride on bikes, skateboards, and all-terrain vehicles; and they get hurt by adults.

This chapter will discuss child health in the national context with the narrowing focus on children with brain injuries. Epidemiology, causes and a definition of brain injury will be provided and outcome data presented which demonstrate why infants and toddlers with brain injury do less well than non-disabled children. The cost of pediatric brain injury to society will be presented with the backdrop of prevention. Finally, the role and development of a pediatric rehabilitation plan will be outlined which includes a specific example.

Child Health in the National Context

Health has become the nation's second largest employer and third largest in consumer spending (Califano, 1986). It is currently near 15% of the Gross National Product. Miracle drugs, genetic engineering, electronics, lasers, and nuclear scanners have been developed to assure us of our seeming birthright, excellent health care.

And yet something is terribly wrong. Despite the vast sums poured into health care, the United States ranks 12th among nations in life expectancy; 21st in the number of deaths of children under age 5; 22nd in infant mortality; and 24th in the percentage of babies born with an adequate birthweight. Among industrialized nations, only the United States and South Africa fail to provide access to health care for all their citizens (Consumer Report, September, 1990). Even more disturbing is the fact that Singapore spends $200 per person on health, has a lower infant mortality, and the same life expectancy as the United States.

There is increasing pressure understandably to curb medical spending in the United States. We are experiencing a form of medical economic Darwinism - medical survival of those with health insurance and an ever widening gap between those with access to health care and those without. At risk in this bipolar medical delivery system between the insured and uninsured, is who suffers how much for how long, and who dies (Capliano, 1986). The problems inherent in this Darwinian system have grave implications for our most vulnerable members, infants and children.

> Children are known to be resilient and adaptable. Children are also known to be vulnerable and easily damaged by social, psychic, and physical traumas and neglect. If children are blighted by failures to meet their need, what are the long and short term costs to society? (Miller, Fine & Adams-Taylor, 1989, p. 2).

How do our nation's health policies and resources fit our smallest citizens? Health policy "may be regarded as the aggregate of principles or themes that prevail in the ways society distributes its resources and power as they relate to the determinants of a population's state of health" (Miller et al., 1989, p. 2).

Considerations of the biological and medical determinants of health have usually dominated health policy which has generally brought us advances in biomedical technology. In manners of health policy we seek medical answers to social problems. This approach is done at great expense but it appears we would rather do this than develop social reforms that might have a more meaningful impact on health status.

> The cost of giving one child all recommended child health preventive services from birth to age 20 is approximately equal to the cost of one day in the hospital. Unfortunately, too often children's health needs are addressed only when they are acutely ill. (Giebink, 1986).

The fact that so few dollars are committed to prevention of childhood disease and injury has grave implications for our society.

Babies are born with low birthweight or intrauterine cerebral injury because of poor access to prenatal care for mothers. Well documented child abuse and neglect continue to increase. Fatalities and injuries from motor vehicle accidents have increased, associated with an increase in recreational driving, often in combination with substance abuse. Gunshot wounds to the head are increasing and reflect even more poignantly our country's emphasis on seeking medical answers to social problems. Children are surviving these accidents because of improved biomedical technology when they shouldn't end up in the Emergency Room in the first place. Nowhere is the lack of attention to prevention of injury more impressive than in the case of infants and children who receive traumatic brain injuries.

Children with Brain Injuries

A tragedy too familiar to the author is the life of a normally developing child suddenly interrupted by an injury to the brain. The injury can be caused by physical trauma such as closed head injuries sustained in automobile, bike and pedestrian accidents; falls; and recreational vehicle accidents (snowmobiles, four-wheelers); open head injuries which are generally sustained by gunshot wounds; and anoxic injuries where the damage to the brain is caused by loss of oxygen as in near drowning and suffocation. In all of these accidents, the common denominator is the same: an injury to a child's brain that will interrupt learning, cause behavior problems, and prevent that child from reaching his or her full potential. The injury will also play havoc with the entire family which, in reality, is as injured as the child.

Traumatic Brain Injury

In this section the epidemiology and categories of traumatic brain injury will be presented and a functional definition provided.

Epidemiology

In childhood and adolescence, accidents are the leading cause of death and disability, and the majority of these deaths and disabilities are due to brain injury (Lehr, 1990). Half of all deaths in childhood, ages 1 to 14, result from accidents (National Center for Health Statistics) and this figure is twice that of cancer and congenital defects combined.

Over one million children receive traumatic brain injuries each year (Lehr, 1990). A more concrete description of annual incidence might be: 66,666 Little League Baseball Teams; or 33,333 second grade classes; or 1,666 graduation classes from a large urban high school.

In recognition of the need for more accurate prevalence figures, the National Pediatric Trauma Registry was established at the Department of Rehabilitation Medicine at Tufts University with a grant from the National Institute on Disability and Rehabilitation Research.

The objective was to create a database on multiple aspects of childhood trauma, including how children are injured, how their treatment is managed in the hospital, and the physical consequences of trauma to the child. The following findings are based on the April, 1991, report on 13,321 injury cases:

> Boys are almost twice as likely as girls to be injured.
> Blunt trauma (closed head injury) continues to be the most frequent injury affecting children.
> Penetrating injuries are increasing due to an increase in gunshot wounds.
> Falls are the most frequent cause of injury, 26%.
> When traffic-related accidents are combined (motor vehicle occupant, pedestrian, motorcycle, bicycle, recreational vehicle), they account for 45% of all injuries.
> The majority of children (97%) survived their brain injury (NIDRR, 1991).

Categories of Injury

The four categories of injury which provide the foundation for clinical management, parent education and prognosis are closed head injury, open head injury, anoxia and infection (Sellars & Vegter, 1993).

Closed Head Injury

The brain is not attached to the skull, and when the head hits or is hit by something, the brain moves around inside the skull. The skull remains intact, but the brain is damaged by the tearing and ripping of the cellular structures. In the same fashion, the brain bruises and bleeds inside the skull.

Damage occurs in both hemispheres of the brain. This damage may be seen as a collection of blood (hematomas) in one or several locations. This blood in the brain causes edema (swelling) and is dangerous. Quick management of this swelling is important in the period immediately following injury because the hard skull does not allow release of this pressure and, unless properly managed, further swelling can occur.

The important characteristic of a closed head injury is that damage occurs across both hemispheres and though sophisticated diagnostic tests are used to assess areas of greatest damage, the best measure of damage is what the child does clinically.

Open Head Injury

In this category of brain injury, the skull is broken or penetrated. For example, the skull can fracture when the head hits the dashboard of a car; a bullet can pierce the skull; or the skull can be crushed by a kicking horse. These open injuries result in bleeding and bruising inside the brain also but often the damage is more localized, contained to one hemisphere.

Anoxia

A severe brain injury can be caused by lack of oxygen to the brain, as is the case when children have respiratory and/or cardiac arrest in near drowning accidents, choking, or status epilepticus, a constant seizuring of the brain. This category results in damage to both hemispheres and prognostically, the long term outcome is typically poor.

Infection

Encephalitis and meningitis are occasional causes of brain injury in children. Encephalitis refers to swelling of the brain due to toxins, infection or tumors. Meningitis refers to swelling of the coverings of the brain, the meninges.

Encephalitis is usually caused by a viral infection and meningitis by a bacterial infection. Sometimes these children have permanent brain damage from the subsequent swelling of the brain (Dodson & Alexander,1986).

With the exception of a very localized, penetrating wound, the diffuse damage seen in the vast majority of children ultimately results in a decrease in brain volume or mass. Over time, the primary injuries of bleeding, bruising, and swelling resolve and the remaining result is less brain mass. This is termed atrophy and is caused by enlarged lateral ventricles which decrease the amount of brain tissue.

Definition

Historically, significant brain injury has been associated with sustained loss of consciousness, but recent research (Boll, 1983) has identified residual cognitive and behavioral deficits following minor head injury, sometimes with no loss of consciousness.

From a purely practical level, it is best to view brain injury on a continuum of severity ranging from no loss of consciousness to death. The definition below is clinical, practical and prognostic.

Brain Injury:

1. A sudden injury to the brain of a child
2. Who has a history of normalcy
3. Which results in a reduction in that child's ability to learn (Sellars & Vegter, 1993).

The history of normalcy can range from a few months in an infant to 17 years in a high school student.

Outcome of Children with Brain Injuries

Much more is known about the outcome of injury in adults than children and research is just beginning in outcome of infants and toddlers. In adults the nature of the brain is a unitary phenomenon, whereas in children it is in a state of constant developmental change. Historically, professionals expected children to do better than adults but research is disputing this paradigm and in fact new research is demonstrating that there is a positive correlation between age at injury and outcome. With infants, toddlers and very young children the outcome is often less good.

This is because of many reasons. Anatomically, in the infant and very young child, the immature skull is thinner, more pliable and more easily transformed by trauma. Also, the developing brain is closer to the brain covering, has a smaller cushioning space and is able to move around more freely. This increases the likelihood of subarachnoid hemorrhages and diffuse injury to nerve fibers.

A study of 51 children (Kriel, Krach & Penser, 1989) compared outcome of children injured before and after six years of age. Children injured after six had better motoric and cognitive outcomes than the younger group. This difference was postulated to be etiological in that some of the children in the youngest group had head injuries secondary to abuse. It is a commonly held belief that these children may have had previous abuse injuries resulting in poorer outcomes.

In a more recent study, Levin et al., (1992) investigated severe head injury in children, experience of the Traumatic Coma Data Bank. Outcome was evaluated in 103 children, 35 of whom were 0 to 4 at the time of their injury. Results indicated mortality was highest and outcome worse in this youngest group.

In a groundbreaking study on outcome of children with prolonged unconsciousness and vegetative states (Kriel, Krach & Jones-Saete, 1993), 60 children were studied who had been unconscious for longer than 90 days. Eight children who died had remained in persistent vegetative states. Most neurological improvement occurred with the first year after injury, although some delayed improvements were observed. Better cognitive and motor outcomes were noted with nonanoxic injuries. The remarkable contrast with adults following acquired brain injury is the significantly longer survival of children. The only children who died had remained in persistent vegetative states.

Persistent Vegetative State

The term "persistent vegetative state" was suggested in 1972 (Jennett & Blum) to describe patients with irreversible brain damage, who on recovery from deep coma pass into a state of seeming wakefulness and reflex responsiveness but do not return to a cognitive state. The term "vegetative" refers to sufficient preservation of the brain stem to sustain the vegetative functions of respiration, circulation and usually eating.

Most all patients recovering from brain injury pass through this stage of vegetative coma, a period of arousal with minimal responses to maximum stimulation. The clinical puzzle is to determine when the child will persist in this condition with no hope for cognitive recovery. As stated previously, children with prolonged anoxia as the cause of their brain damage have a much more guarded prognosis related to achieving cognitive outcome.

In cases of nonanoxic injury, twenty six children with traumatic injury (Kriel, Krach & Sheehan, 1988) were studied and functional outcome correlated with degree of cerebral atrophy on CT Scan. The children were all in a coma for greater than 90 days. Six remained in a persistent vegetative state two or more years post injury, one died, and 19 regained consciousness. The children who regained consciousness continued with significant motoric and cognitive deficits.

Infants Born with Brain Injury

Much of this chapter has been devoted to infants and children who sustain a traumatic brain insult after birth. There are of course infants who receive brain injuries before, during or immediately after birth. Like traumatic injury, this brain insult is nonprogressive and is generally termed Cerebral Palsy. From a purely pragmatic, clinical view, the main distinguishing difference between these cases of congenital and acquired brain injury is the lack of history of normalcy in babies born with brain damage.

The impairments in movement, speech, language, sensory status and cognition are similar. The longevity of these impairments is greater and family adjustment issues different.

Causes of cerebral palsy include unidentifiable problems during intrauterine development (infections, biochemical abnormalities), birth difficulties resulting in anoxia to the brain and low infant birth weight.

More than 90% of children with cerebral palsy live to adulthood, although the life expectancy of severely involved individuals is significantly less than that of the general population, often because of respiratory complications (Evans, Evans, & Alberman, 1991).

Ever increasing efforts to help high-risk babies to survive at birth and in the newborn period are necessary. There are many healthy survivors of these efforts but also the disadvantage - a slowly increasing group of children who have sustained brain injuries. Most epidemiologic studies from industrialized countries show a rise in the childhood prevalence of cerebral palsy, largely because of the increasing contribution of children of low and very low birthweight to its prevalence (Bhushan, Paneth & Kiely, 1993).

Regardless of when the brain damage occurred, before, during or after birth, the collection of disability symptoms are very similar. Thus, in forensic cases the role of a pediatric specialist in brain injury is very important.

THE COST

It is difficult to find specific data relative to the economic burden of children being injured. Often the accident robs many of them of economic independence, not to mention the unbelievable cost of rehabilitation. As a backdrop to this section, the following cases are presented which represent typical scenarios of pediatric rehabilitation to the author.

John, 7 years of age, received a suffocation anoxic injury when he fell into a construction hole and was covered by dirt. He is unable to control the severe spasticity of his body, cannot speak, and cannot feed himself. He is very alert and smiles to jokes but it is not possible to assess his cognition. Five months of rehabilitation costs to date are $103,169. This does not include his acute medical cost covering 4 weeks. It is projected John will continue to be wheelchair dependent and unable to speak the rest of his life.

George is 7 years of age and received a severe head injury in a pedestrian/car accident. He has a tracheostomy and a feeding tube in his stomach. He responds to tone of voice and sensory stimulation. He cannot follow commands and is wheelchair dependent. His single mother is unable to care for him in the home and the hospital is attempting to place him in a nursing home. There are very few facilities in the country for children who are dependent in all cares. Nine months of rehabilitative cost to date is $248,136.

In 1987, Congress asked the National Highway Traffic Safety Administration to measure the cost of injury and associated disability. Results were staggering and implications for prevention efforts evident. One of every four U.S. residents is injured every year. This amounts to 57 million people; younger persons and males are the most affected; and for every person killed, there are 16 hospitalized. The lifetime cost of these injuries is an estimated $158 billion dollars, derived using the human capital approach. This method estimates losses resulting from death or disability by calculating lost productivity. Direct costs, in the form of medical and related services, make up 29% of the lifetime costs.

These injuries cause private grief but do not necessarily produce only a private burden. The costs are great to our society. Airbags, bike helmets, seat belts and raising the driving age one year could effectively reduce the mortality and morbidity of brain injuries in children. Until prevention efforts improve, it seems we will continue to find medical solutions to social problems.

Pediatric Rehabilitation: Planning and Management

The academic background presented for this chapter may be considered exhaustive when the purpose is to present the case for Rehabilitation and Long Term Planning in pediatric cases by a specialist in children with brain injuries. It is the author's intention, by way of this academic background, to make it very evident that babies, toddlers and children are not the same as adults with brain injury. They are in process of development when they are injured and do not have the luxury of a history of previous learning from which to draw. What they are already able to do when they are injured is so incredibly crucial to their outcome. You can see the tragedy of injured babies within this developmental paradigm.

Qualifications of a Pediatric Forensic Specialist

A pediatric forensic specialist should meet the following academic, clinical and social qualifications.

The academic background should include a Doctor of Philosophy Degree in Health or Rehabilitation, respected publications, academic and/or clinical faculty appointments, and evidence of lectures and courses present nationally and internationally in the specialty area of children with brain injuries.

Clinically, the specialist should be actively and intensively engaged in the clinical treatment of these children and their families. The credibility of this specialist is best augmented by a clinical practice because estimates of current needs and prognostic predictions come more fluently from a clinical specialist.

Socially, the specialist should be on community boards and committees which function in an advocacy capacity for the specific disability group of children with brain injuries. Volunteerism reflects commitment, care and citizenship.

Finally, and perhaps most importantly, this person must be academically, clinically and socially grounded in pediatric disabilities to present information confidently and fluently. (Elliot, 1993)

Rehabilitation Life Care Planning and Case Management: Coordinated Pediatric Care

First and foremost, the role of the Pediatric Rehabilitation Specialist is education. The initial task is to determine the consequences of the injury and develop a rehabilitation plan to maximize that child's potential. The substrata are always the careful analysis of the disability, the projection of functional outcome, and a thoughtful, realistic view of projected life time needs.

Such specialists are useful for consultation with plaintiff and defense attorneys in catastrophic cases, coordination of the myriad of services often needed to allow consistently high quality care for the child, education of lay persons about pediatric disabilities and ongoing evaluation of service delivery to the child. (Elliot, 1993)

Cost containment is best and most realistically obtained when the right amount of services are provided by pediatric experts at just the right time in the child's development. This principle maximizes functional outcome which, in turn, reduces longer term, more expensive costs when treatment is not provided or not provided well. The goal is to effectively reduce the child's long term need for support by providing it when it counts. This is true cost containment and it allows the child maximum service when appropriate.

The Rehabilitation Specialist in pediatric cases reviews all medical records, may evaluate the child personally, evaluates the opposing expert's recommendations, and acts as liaison between the rehabilitation and legal professions and the family. The actual rehabilitation plan becomes a graphic extension for attorneys, courts, parents and payors of a careful, detailed analysis of the child's current disabilities and projected needs. It is what the specialist believes to be an effective utilization of financial resources which will enable that child to become the most functional adult possible within the realistic constraints of the brain injury.

Development of the Rehabilitation and Life Care Plan

Purpose

Rehabilitation Life Care Planning looks beyond the acute care needs caused by injury to project the effects that injury will have on the child's current status and future functioning as an adult. The specialist must have a knowledge of evaluation, therapeutic equipment, drugs, medical care, environmental adaptations, and possible residential needs that may develop over the child's lifetime and have access to information on their cost, goals, frequency and duration (Deutsch & Sawyer, 1985).

Specific Parameters

The specific parameters of a pediatric plan are often organized into the following categories.

I. Medical Care
   A. Medical Evaluation: Routine medical management is critical to prevent very costly medical complications and assist in functional changes. These evaluations may include Physiatry, Pediatrics, Otolaryngology, Pediatric and eventually Adult Neurology, Audiology and Dental/ Orthodontic Evaluations.
   B. Developmental Evaluations: Periodic developmental assessments are done to maximize independence by providing specific therapy recommendations to school staff who are not as familiar with children with brain injuries. These recommendations are also provided to Personal Care Attendants and, of course, parents. They may include psychological assessment, speech pathology, physical and

occupational therapy, neuropsychological assessment and possibly a driving evaluation.

C. Medications and Supplies:
   1. Medications: Often babies and children with brain injuries receive medication to control seizures, reduce tone or aid digestion. Costs must be included.
   2. Supplies: Supplies often include diapers, feeding, respiratory supplies and standard medical supply support.

II. Equipment: Durable medical equipment is often required through a child's lifetime.

A. Mobility: This equipment category includes wheelchairs, adapted bicycles, walkers, safe care seats, and positioning and home therapy aids.

B. Aids to Independence: This equipment is used to assist the child to be as independent as possible in eating, bathing, dressing and toileting.

C. Learning Equipment: This category includes augmentative communication equipment if indicated cognitively, a home computer and educational software to maximize learning and often provide appropriate writing adaptations for schoolwork.

III. Therapeutic Support: Direct therapeutic support for children in speech, physical and occupational therapy is often recommended to augment therapy provided in the school system and/or enable the child to receive therapy through the summer at developmentally appropriate stages.

IV. Home Modifications: If the child will be wheelchair dependent, home modifications are recommended so the home environment can be safely accessible to the child.

V. Car Modifications: Once again, if the child is wheelchair dependent and, depending on his/her ability to transfer, a van equipped with a lift may be recommended for transportation. This is recommended when the child is unable to transfer to a safe, adapted care seat in a regular automobile.

VI. Long Term Care and Treatment: This category requires a careful judgement of future status. Recommendations can be provided about the child's future ability to live independently; with minimal assistance in the form of Personal Care Attendants; a group home with professional assistance; or a Long Term Care Facility because of profound disabilities.

This categorical list is not all inclusive and certainly each case is unique. It does, however, provide major categories of care and cost projection.

Predicting Outcome: Recovery Versus Development

As mentioned previously, one of the greatest challenges in pediatrics is projecting disability when the child is in a state of developmental change as part of neurological maturation. This can be very difficult because often there is not objective pre-injury data of intellectual status. This is particularly true if the child has not yet attended school.

The very best way to predict with some sense of accuracy is to carefully look at all developmental testing since injury to find the child's learning rate. For example, if a 3 year old child with a traumatic brain injury receives developmental levels of a 2 year old at discharge from acute rehabilitation, and scores of 2 years, 8 months one year later it looks clinically like this child is cognitively developing at approximately 2/3s of her chronological age. This developmental rate is correlated with an Intelligence Quotient of approximately 70, or a mild delay in intelligence. At age 12 it is suggested her developmental levels would be near an 8 year level. The greater longevity of test scores, the more accurate the prediction.

Cost Containment: Is Therapy Ever Over?

Another very difficult issue in projecting costs is what efficacy direct therapy will have on a child's functional independence. All professionals will agree that direct therapy is crucial in the early years following injury but is there ever a point when therapy is not indicated any longer? I think so.

Therapies that concentrate on preventing complications of muscle contractures may be needed at least in a evaluative format through a child's lifetime with actual exercises provided by a paraprofessional. Speech pathology and occupational therapy directed toward language and visual perceptual changes may likely outlive their usefulness as the child matures. Clearly there are critical stages in development when therapy should be maximized. One of these stages is imitation and when a child begins this stage, aggressive cognitively based therapies are indicated. It is the author's belief that often direct therapy takes the place of encouragement of development in the more natural milieu of community recreational activities, the home and school. Developmental and cognitive progress occurs in more natural environments with peers and family. It is, however, a common belief among parents and some professionals that therapy is the only catalyst for change.

Collateral Sources of Support of Children

There are many sources of collateral funds for children with disabilities, particularly children in low income families. These of course include health programs such as Medicaid and Medicare, Social Security benefits, and special programs related to camping, leisure and recreation, and transportation. However, the most important collateral support for children is education.

The Education of the Handicapped Act has been renamed to Individuals with Disabilities Education Act (IDEA) or P.L. 101-476. Eligibility for special education now includes children with traumatic brain injury. Direct therapy services are provided to assist the child in obtaining educational or instructional goals. For example, the hospital occupational therapist may work on arm strengthening while the school occupational therapist may work on adapting a computer so the child can do homework on a keyboard with their nondominant, uninjured hand.

IDEA also includes provision for transition services and planning. These services are to include any instruction that will assist in post-secondary education, vocational training, integrated employment, continuing and adult education, adult services, independent living and community integration.

It is very important for the Pediatric Rehabilitation Specialist to understand the school system in the child's community to assist in obtaining efficient use of this very supportive collateral source for children with disabling conditions.

A Pediatric Rehabilitation and Life Care Plan

Case Background

A synopsis of an actual case may be helpful to conclude this section on Pediatric Rehabilitation Life Care Planning. Obviously, distinguishing characteristics, name and location, have been changed to protect the child. The medical and developmental summaries are a very brief synopsis.

Olivia was one year, ten months of age when she received a brain injury in an automobile accident. She had a left frontal-temporal skull fracture and a penetrating injury to the left temporal area. These injuries were treated acutely, and Olivia spent four months as an inpatient in a pediatric rehabilitation facility.

Discharge testing from that facility indicated Olivia was developmentally at an 18 to 24 month level, chronological age of 27 months.

She returned home and entered a community based Early Education Preschool Program with supportive assistance in speech, occupational and physical therapy.

At the time the author reviewed her case and conducted an

evaluation, Olivia was three and a half years of age. Her presenting problems were a dense right hemiplegia. She was unable to walk without assistance but did scoot on her buttocks for mobility. She did not use her right hand functionally. Her cognitive and language development was at a two to two and a half year level.

It was projected Olivia would be able to walk short distances with a walker but would require a wheelchair for long distances. It was projected her mental development would progress at a rate which would be considered moderate retardation. It was projected she could engage in supportive employment and live in a group home with other physically and mentally disabled adults in her community.

Though her injury and concomitant disabilities were considered moderate, it was projected her life time functional abilities would be reasonable. Pragmatically, this would mean Olivia would live with adults with similar disabilities, work in a supervised setting and be semi-independent in her community.

Table 7.1 presents an outline of the recommendations made in Olivia's case for rehabilitation during her developmental years and extended support and supervision throughout her life.

TABLE 7.1 *Rehabilitation and Life Care Plan*

Recommendation	Frequency/Duration	Cost Estimate
I. Medical Care		
A. Medical Evaluations		
1. Pediatrician	2 times/year to age 16	130/year to age 16
2. Physiatrist	2 times/year to life expectancy	240/year
3. Pediatric Neurology	1 time/year to age 19	125/year to age 19
4. Adult Neurology	1 time/year, age 19 to life expectancy	125/year, age 19 to life expectancy
5. Audiology	2 times/year to age 16	147/year to age 16
6. Scoliosis Profile	1 time/year to age 16	291/year to age 16
B. Developmental Evaluations		
1. Educational Psychology	1 time/year to age 21	N/A: Included in annual educational evaluation

Continued

TABLE 7.1 *Rehabilitation and Life Care Plan, continued*

Recommendation	Frequency/Duration	Cost Estimate
2. Speech Pathology	2 times/year to age 21; 1 time/year, age 22 to life expectancy	140/year to age 21; then included in facility per diem
3. Physical Therapy	2 times/year to life expectancy	180/year to age 21; then included in facility per diem
4. Occupational Therapy	2 times/year to life expectancy	140/year to age 21; then included in facility per diem
C. Medications and Supplies		
1. Tegretol	100 mg/4 times day	324/year to age 21; then included in facility per diem
2. Large Diapers	To age 6	747/year to age 6
II. Equipment		
A. Mobility		
1. Wheelchair: pediatric with one arm drive	1 time/5 years to age 11	2,700/5 years to age 11
2. Wheelchair: adult with one arm drive	1 time/5 years, age 16 to life expectancy	2,000/5 years, ages 16 to life expectancy
3. Pediatric walker with right forearm attach.	1 time/5 years to age 11	450/5 years to age 11
4. Adult walker with right forearm attach.	1 time/5 years, age 16 to life expectancy	250/5 years, ages 16 to life expectancy
5. Lapboard	1 time/5 years to life	60/5 years to life expectancy
6. Hand drive trike	1 time only at age 6	680
7. Adult trike	1 time only at age 12	365
B. Aids to Independence		
1. Therapy Ball	1 time/5 years to age 15	47/5 years to age 15
2. Child's Bath Support	1 time only	295
3. Hand Held Shower	1 time only	37.95
4. Easy Care Shower Chair	1 time only at age 12	355
5. Safety Grab Bar and Bathing	1 time only	21
6. Right AFO	1 time/year to age 16; then 1 time/3 years to life expectancy	525/year to age 16; then 525 every 3 years to life expectancy
7. Right Hand Splint	1 time/year to age 16; then 1 time/3 years to life expectancy	53/year to age 16; then 53 every 3 years to life expectancy
8. Adapted Eating Utensils	1 time/5 years	36.75/5 years

Continued

TABLE 7.1 *Rehabilitation and Life Care Plan, continued*

Recommendation	Frequency/Duration	Cost Estimate
C. Learning Equipment		
1. IBM Compatible or Macintosh Computer	1 time/10 years to life expectancy	1,000/10 years
2. Ancillary Computer Equipment	1 time/10 years to life expectancy	5,00/10 years
3. Educational Software	1 time/3 years to life expectancy	1,000 the first year; then 500 every 3 years
III. <u>Therapy Support</u>		
A. Speech Therapy	3 times weekly to age 21	N/A: Costs provided by school under public law PL101.476
B. Occupational Therapy	2-3 times weekly to age 21	N/A: Costs provided by school under public law PL101.476
C. Physical Therapy	2-3 times/weekly to age 21	N/A: Costs provided by school under public law PL101.476
D. Supplemental Speech Therapy	2 times/week in summer to age 10	1,200/year to age 10
E. Supplemental Occupational Therapy	2 times/week in summer to age 10	1,200/year to age 10
F. Supplemental Physical Therapy	2 times/week in summer to age 10	1,200/year to age 10
IV. <u>Home/Facility Care</u>		
Recommendations to Age 21		
1. Home Care Aid	2 hours/day to age 7; then 4 hours/day ages 7-21	5,840/year to age 7; then 11,680/year ages 7-21 (Based on 8/hour)
2. Home Care Manager	10 hours/month to age 21	3,000/year to age 21 (Based on 25/hour)
3. Miscellaneous Costs (FICA; Accounting; Payroll, etc.)	N/A	1326/year to age 7; then 2,202/year to age 21 (Based on 15% of gross payroll)
	Total Home Care	10,166/year to age 7; 16,882/year ages 7-21
After Age 21		
1. Specialized Neurologic Residential Facility with coordinated day program	24 hour/day care, treatment and supervision to life expectancy	36,945/year to life expectancy

Continued

TABLE 7.1 *Rehabilitation and Life Care Plan, continued*

Recommendation	Frequency/Duration	Cost Estimate
2. Case Manager	2 hours/month	1,560/year to life expectancy
V. Architectural Renovations		
1. Home Modification for wheelchair accessibility	1 time only to permanent dwelling	20,000-30,000, 1 time only

CONCLUSION

Every chapter eventually arrives by way of conclusion to the main point. It has been my major intent to present the case that infants, toddlers and young children with brain injuries are very different than adults. Their special needs require the services of a pediatric specialist for Rehabilitation and Life Care Planning.

Children are not little adults. Evaluation of their status and projection of their future requires the thoughtful objectivity of a specialist in pediatric rehabilitation.

And by way of final conclusion, whenever I write or lecture I always feel bound by my clinical experience to present a plea for continued efforts on behalf of protecting these young children of ours. Air bags, bicycle helmets, and seat belts seem like such an easy solution, but our society continues to place the dollars in the trauma and post trauma care of these children. When private grief and shattered development are considered, this does seem an unusual prioritizing of dollars.

If people of science could find the time and the courage to think honestly and critically over their situation and the paths before them, and if they would act accordingly, the possibilities for asensible and satisfactory solution would be considerably improved.

Albert Einstein

We wish for your children safety in all things.

References

Bhushan, V., Paneth, N., Kelly, J. (June, 1993). Impact of improved survival of very low birth weight infants on recent secular trends in the prevalence of cerebral palsy. *Pediatrics*, 91(6), 1094-1100.

Boll, T. (1983). Minor head injury in children- Out of sight but not out of mind. *Journal of Clinical Psychology,* 12(1), 74-80.

Burke, W. (1994). The rehabilitation expert: Analysis and management of brain injury and other neurologic disorders. In Burke, W.H. (Ed.). *The Handbook of Forensic Rehabilitation.* Houston, TX: HDI.

Capliano, J. (1986). *Health Care Revolution.* New York, NY: Touchstone.

Crisis in health insurance: Can you afford to get sick? (August, 1990). *Consumer Reports,* 533-549.

Deutsch, P. & Sawyer, H. (1985). *A Guide to Rehabilitation.* New York, NY: Matthew Bender.

Dodson, F. & Alexander, A. (1986). *Your Child: Birth to Age 6.* New York, NY: Simon and Schuster.

Elliot, T. (1993). Life care plans: the legal perspective. *The Neurolaw Letter*, 2 (11).

Evans, P., Evans, S. & Alberman, E. (December, 1990). Cerebral palsy: Why we must plan for survival. *Archives of Disease in Childhood,* 65, 1329-1333.

Giebink, G. (Fall, 1986). Unpublished paper presented at the American Academy of Pediatrics. *Minnesota Pediatrician.*

Jennett, B. & Plum, F., (1972). Persistent vegetative state: A syndrome in search of a name. *Lancet,* 4, 743-747.

Kriel, R., Krach, L. & Jones-Saete, C. (September-October, 1993). Outcome of children with prolonged unconsciousness and vegetative states. *Pediatric Neurology,* 9(5), 362-368.

Kriel, R., Krach, L. & Penser, L. (1989).Closed head injury in children: Comparison of children younger and older than 6 years of age. *Pediatric Neurology,* 5(5), 296-300.

Kriel, R., Krach, L. & Sheehan, M., (1988). Pediatric closed head injury: Outcome following prolonged unconsciousness. *Archives of Physical Medicine and Rehabilitation,* 69, 678-681.

Lehr, E., (1990). *Psychological Management of Traumatic Brain Injuries in Children.* Rockville, MD: Aspen.

Levin, H., Aldrich, E., Saydjan, C., Eisenberg, H., Foulkes, M., Bellefleur, M., Luerssen, T., Jane, J., Marmaneu, A., Marshall, L. & Young, H. (Sept. 1992). Severe head injury in children: Experience of the Traumatic Coma Data Bank. *Neurosurgery,* 32(3), 435-444.

Miller, C., Fine, A. & Adams-Taylor, J. (1989). *Monitoring Children's Health: Key Indicators.* (2nd ed.). Washington, D.C.: American Public Health Association.

Sellars, C. (Fall, 1992). Children with brain injuries: A costly tragedy. *Minnesota Trial Lawyer's Magazine.*

Sellars, C. & Vegter, C. (1993). *Pediatric Brain Injury: A Practical Resource.* Tucson, AZ: Communication Skill Builders.

Carole Wedel Sellars, Ph.D. - Director of Pediatric Brain Injury

Dr. Sellars is the founder and coordinator of the Pediatric Brain Injury Program at Gillette Children's Hospital, St. Paul, Minnesota. Dr. Sellars is a certified speech and language pathologist and is a member of the adjunct clinical faculty of the University of Minnesota. She was a founding member of the Minnesota Head Injury Association and served on the Board of Directors from 1987-1993. Dr. Sellars recently co-authored a text entitled *Pediatric Brain Injury: A Practical Resource*, and is currently completing a book on infants and toddlers with brain injury.

William H. Burke, Ph.D.

See page 52

8

THE NEUROLOGIC EXAMINATION IN FORENSIC EVALUATION

Sheldon Margulies, M.D., J.D.

Brain injuries are the most devastating injuries to the human body but they are also, ironically, the most difficult to diagnose and quantify. Physiatrists, psychologists, internists, even chiropractors render opinions about brain damage, but clearly, the specialists most qualified to diagnose brain damage are neurologists and neurosurgeons.

The purpose of this chapter is to introduce basic neuroanatomy and neurophysiology, explain some of the common neurologic tests, and emphasize the importance of the neurologic exam.

Brain Anatomy and Physiology

Brain Stem

The anatomy of the brain is best understood by beginning with the brain stem, the most primitive part of the brain. The brain stem controls functions shared by all animals: consciousness, eye movements, facial movements, facial sensation, swallowing, breathing, blood pressure, and temperature regulation. The bottom end of the brain stem exits the base of the skull through a large hole called the foramen magnum. This is the point at which the brain stem becomes the upper end of the spinal cord.

The most important function of the brain stem is to generate "electricity" for a "light bulb" screwed into each hemisphere.

Fortunately, being so deep in the brain the brain stem is well protected. There have, however, been cases in which patients have suffered direct damage to the brain stem, rendering them comatose for months or even years, and then woken up normal. This would not happen if the patient were rendered comatose by a traumatic injury to both hemispheres.

Cerebellum

Our ability to walk and use our limbs in a coordinated fashion is governed by three completely separate motor control systems in the brain: the cerebellum, the basal ganglia, and the corticospinal tract. The cerebellum sits behind the brain stem and controls our balance and coordination. Cerebellar malfunction causes ataxia, the best example being alcohol intoxication which produces truncal ataxia. Truncal ataxia is tested by having the patient walk a straight line, heel to toe. Ataxia of the arms causes an intention tremor: the hand shakes as it nears its target. Such patients cannot drink from a full cup without spilling its contents.

Thalamus

Resting atop the brain stem are the left and right thalamus. All sensory signals destined for the brain must stop in the thalamus before being allowed to enter consciousness. On instructions from the cerebral cortex, the thalamus decides which sensory signals are important enough to interrupt the concentration (or sleep) of the cerebral cortex. Certain parts of the thalamus are also vital for memory.

Basal Ganglia

In the upper part of the brain stem and just above the brain stem is the second motor control system called the basal ganglia, composed of islands of nerve cells ("ganglia") deep in the brain ("basal"). The basal ganglia control the speed and spontaneity of our movements. The best known basal ganglia illness is Parkinson's disease: patients become immobile and rigid, and walk with a slow shuffling gait.

Corticospinal Tract

Every nerve cell, or neuron, has a cell body and an axon. Nerve cell bodies stain gray and the axons white, so wherever there is a collection of nerve cell bodies the brain stains gray, and wherever the axons run the brain stains white, hence the terms gray matter and white matter. The cerebral cortex is a rind of gray matter — nerve cell bodies — over the entire surface of the brain.

White matter is a thick, dense network of axons (neurologic "wires") carrying signals to and from the cerebral cortex. The reason the basal ganglia are islands of gray matter amidst a sea of white matter deep in the brain is that in prehistoric animals the basal ganglia used to be the most advanced gray matter structure of the brain. Because of the need for a more advanced motor system to control limbs and fingers, evolution (or God) developed the more advanced cerebral cortex over the surface of the brain with a thick bed of white matter axons below the cortex, leaving the basal ganglia buried deep within the white matter.

Nerves work by sending an electrical signal from a nerve cell body in the gray matter down its axon to terminate on the next nerve cell. When the electrical signal reaches the terminus of the axon, neurotransmitters are squirted out to stimulate the next nerve. The neurotransmitters are manufactured in the cell body and transported down the axon. In mild head injury, this axonal transport system is stunned. It takes hours or days, sometimes months, for axonal transport to be restarted during which the patient may feel fuzzy and forgetful.

Within the white matter of the brain is one especially important tract called the corticospinal tract. Whenever we want to move a limb, two nerves are needed: an upper motor neuron and a lower motor neuron. The upper motor neuron carries instructions from the motor strip in the cerebral cortex downward through the brain stem into the spinal cord. The instructions are then relayed to the lower motor neuron which exits the spinal cord through nerve roots and then travels via peripheral nerves to the muscle. Upper motor neurons from the motor strip are bundled together into a tract called the corticospinal tract.

Damage to the corticospinal tract causes five important neurologic signs. The most commonly recognized one is hemiplegia (paralysis of an arm and leg). Other signs of corticospinal tract dysfunction include spasticity (stiffness), slowing of fine dexterity, hyperreflexia, and Babinski sign (upgoing great toe when the sole is scraped). Both the spasticity of corticospinal tract dysfunction and the rigidity of basal ganglia dysfunction cause stiffness of the limbs, but spasticity is easily distinguishable from rigidity on neurologic exam.

Lobes of Each Hemisphere

The brain is divided into a left and right hemisphere. Each hemisphere is in turn divided into four lobes: temporal, frontal, occipital, and parietal. The largest lobe is the frontal lobe, extending back to the middle of the skull. Lateral to the frontal lobe lies the temporal lobe (behind the temple), separated from the frontal lobe by a large cleft called the Sylvian fissure. Behind the frontal and temporal lobes is the parietal lobe. The occipital lobes occupy the rear of each hemisphere.

Temporal Lobe

Memory is divided into short-term and long-term, short-term generally referring to the ability to lay down new memories, and long-term referring to the ability to retrieve established memories. The ability to recognize established memories from a list is a third type of memory. Short-term memory is controlled by the temporal lobes, the left temporal lobe favoring verbal memories, the right temporal lobe favoring non-verbal memories (designs and shapes). The critical structure in the temporal lobe responsible for laying down new memories is the hippocampus and overlying entorhinal cortex.

The hippocampus is also part of a very old system in the brain called the limbic system where emotions are experienced. Emotions and memories are connected for a good reason — so that we would remember the emotionally charged events in our lives.

Sitting in the middle fossa with its nose against the sphenoid wing, which acts like a bony "windshield", the temporal lobe is vulnerable to being smacked against the sphenoid wing in frontal trauma. The resulting hippocampal damage can seriously impair short term memory function.

Frontal Lobe

The frontal lobe is also vulnerable to traumatic injury by being smacked up against the frontal bone, injuring the top of the frontal lobe and scraping the inferior surface of the frontal lobe along the rough and irregular floor of the anterior fossa.

Damage to the superior surface of the frontal lobe impairs executive function. Patients lose the ability to solve problems by generating hypotheses, shifting one's thoughts rapidly between hypotheses, planning strategies to rule out the hypotheses, and keeping information in temporary memory storage for use in solving problems. Frontal lobe patients also have problems remembering where and when they first encountered the memory. Their ability to recognize memories from a list or lay down new memories remains intact. Depression is common when the superior frontal tip of the left hemisphere is injured. The Wisconsin Card Sort Test is touted to be a good test of superior frontal lobe damage.

Damage to the inferior frontal lobe causes changes in personality. Patients lose their initiative and conscientiousness and control of their emotions, becoming outspoken, irritable, tactless, and euphoric.

Damage to the medial frontal lobe, especially the cingulate gyrus, causes apathy. The major neuropsychological deficit demonstrated in patients with medial frontal lobe lesions is failure of response inhibition on go/no go tests

The cingulate gyrus is a very primitive area of the cerebral cortex, connected to the even older subcortical "limbic" system controlling our emotions. The limbic system begins in the temporal lobes and arches via the fornix into the inferior frontal regions and hypothalamus. The hypothalamus is the source for our involuntary responses to emotional situations — blushing, sweating, hair standing on end, pupillary dilation, rise in heart rate, rise in respiratory rate, diarrhea, erections, etc. The hypothalamus "expresses" our emotions via the sympathetic nervous system which travels from the hypothalamus down the brain stem into the spinal cord, and from there to the peripheral nervous system.

Occipital Lobe

The occipital lobes receive and assemble visual information from the retina. Retinal images travel back to the brain in the optic nerve. The optic nerves join each other at the optic chiasm where signals from the medial half of each retina cross to the opposite side. The net result is that the bundles of visual fibers exiting the optic chiasm — the left and right optic tracts — carry signals from the left or right half of the visual world of each eye. The optic tracts wrap around the upper brain stem, ending up in the occipital lobes where the retinal signals are assembled into visual images. Damage to the left occipital lobe causes blindness to the right of midline in each eye, and vice-versa.

Parietal Lobe

It is rare for mild head injury patients to complain of parietal lobe symptoms, perhaps because the parietal lobes are not rounded lobes thrust against the skull as is the case with frontal and temporal lobe injuries.

The parietal lobes are the sensory lobes. Based on input from the skin, the eyes (via the occipital lobes), the ears (via the temporal lobes), and other sensory organs, the parietal lobes assemble and then recognize the shapes and patterns of objects. The right parietal lobe (more than the left) also formulates a mental map of our surroundings, so that patients with right parietal lesions become easily lost in their surroundings, lose the ability to construct simple designs, and get confused over the "topology" of clothing making it difficult for them get dressed.

Membranes In and Around the Brain

Between the two hemispheres is a rigid baffle called the falx. Lateral impacts to the head slap the hemispheres against the falx, making lateral head trauma more injurious than front-to-back trauma.

Delicately laid over the surface of the cerebral cortex is a gossamer-thin membrane called the arachnoid. All structures beneath the arachnoid — the cerebrospinal fluid, the brain, and the arteries and veins supplying the brain — are, by definition, "subarachnoid." Any bleeding beneath the arachnoid, for example, is a subarachnoid hemorrhage. One common example is a cerebral contusion (bruise), which leaks a small amount of blood into the subarachnoid space. The CAT scan is quite good at detecting subarachnoid blood, even better than the MRI.

Encasing the arachnoid is a leathery membrane called the dura. Blood clots that form under the dura are called subdural hematomas and those outside the dura, epidural hematomas. Epidural hematomas are far more dangerous than subdural hematomas because epidural hematomas result from a hemorrhaging artery under high pressure, while subdural hematomas result from a hemorrhaging vein under low pressure. The most common site for an epidural hematoma is over the temporal lobe where the temporal bone is quite thin and easily fractured. The fractured bone tears the middle meningeal artery running epidurally along the inside of the temporal bone.

Cerebral Arteries

The brain is supplied by two major arteries: the carotids, which supply the front of the brain, and the vertebrals, which supply the back of the brain. The carotid arteries run alongside the trachea while the vertebrals travel deep in the neck in a series of bony rings alongside the vertebral bodies.

Once inside the skull, the internal carotid artery divides into the anterior, middle, and posterior cerebral arteries to supply the frontal, temporal, parietal, and occipital lobes. The two vertebral arteries join in front of the brain stem to form a single basilar artery which supplies the brain stem and cerebellum. The top end of the basilar artery is joined by the posterior cerebrals to supply the occipital lobes.

In whiplash injuries the carotids and vertebrals can be stretched suddenly causing bleeding within the arterial wall, called arterial dissection. The whiplash can be from such "benign" things as sneezing vigorously or chiropractic manipulation. The danger of dissection is thrombosis of the artery, causing a stroke.

Headaches following head injuries are usually vascular headaches, i.e., migraine. One, still useful, way to view migraine is that arteries supplying the brain constrict for a brief period followed by painful dilatation of arteries in the scalp. If the constrictive phase is severe enough, the brain can be deprived of blood. Depending on which artery is in spasm, the patient can experience difficulty thinking, word finding difficulties, visual loss, double vision, dizziness, numbness, weakness, ataxia, and incoordination.

Cerebral Veins

The two most important veins in the brain are the cavernous sinus and superior sagittal sinus. (Veins carry blood back to the heart; arteries carry blood away from the heart.) The cavernous sinus, located in front of the brain stem and behind the upper cheek, drains blood from the eye and face. Any infection on the face, including pimples, can shed bacteria into the cavernous sinus and cause a life-threatening illness called septic cavernous sinus thrombosis — hence the term "triangle of death" for the central facial area.

The superior sagittal sinus arches along the inner surface of the skull from the frontal region to the occiput. At the bony protuberance of the occiput (which you can feel on your own skull), the superior sagittal sinus splits into two horizontal veins, called the internal jugular veins, which descend through the neck (next to the carotid arteries) to the heart.

Ventricles and Cerebrospinal Fluid

The brain is a hollow structure. The hollow complex of internal chambers, called the ventricles, contains cerebrospinal fluid which circulates from the ventricles out onto the surface of the brain and down along the spinal cord. Cerebrospinal fluid exits the skull by being absorbed through tiny drain sites embedded in veins lining the inner surface of the skull.

When the flow of cerebrospinal fluid is obstructed anywhere along its course, the fluid dams up and enlarges the ventricles, a condition called hydrocephalus. Trauma to the brain can cause hydrocephalus when a cerebral contusion leaks blood into the spinal fluid, clogging up the drain sites. Three symptoms typically develop in hydrocephalus: confusion (from pressure on the cerebral cortex), stiffness of the gait (pyramidal tracts), and urinary incontinence (upper motor neurons controlling the bladder).

Skull

At birth the skull is made up of a number of bony plates resting atop the dura and brain, much like the geologic plates on the surface of the Earth. The skull plates are free to float until about age 10-12 years when they fuse to form a single, rigid skull bone. The inner surface of the skull is smooth, except for the inferior frontal region where there are grooves and small protuberances. This roughened area of the skull can damage the undersurface of the frontal lobes if the head impact is severe enough to cause the frontal lobes to slide along the skull surface.

Another important area of the skull is the middle fossa where the temporal lobes lie. The front of each middle fossa is made up of a bone called the sphenoid wing, which arches up in front of the temporal lobe. In serious head trauma, the tips of the temporal lobes can be smacked against the sphenoid wings, causing temporal lobe damage.

Brain Physiology

Different areas of the brain control tend to control rather specific functions. Speech, for example, is controlled by structures in the left hemisphere abutting the Sylvian fissure, and vision is controlled by the occipital lobes. For many functions, however, like attention span, memory, reasoning, judgment, and emotions, localization is much less clear because more than one area of the brain participates.

Vision

The best understood function of the cerebral cortex is vision. Retinal images travel back to the brain in the optic nerve. The optic nerves join each other at the optic chiasm in order for signals from the medial half of each retina to cross to the opposite side. The net result is that the bundles of visual fibers exiting the optic chiasm — the left and right optic tracts — carry signals from the left or right half of the visual world of each eye. The optic tracts wrap around the upper brain stem, ending up in the occipital lobes where the retinal signals are assembled into visual images

Lesions of the optic nerve cause five neurologic signs: impaired visual acuity, visual field defects, poor pupillary reaction to light, impaired color vision, and ophthalmologic abnormalities of the optic disc (the tip of the optic nerve plugging into the back of the eyeball). Damage to, say, the left occipital lobe causes blindness to the right of midline in each eye.

Visuomotor complaints involve outgoing signals from the brain — primarily the brain stem. Because the visuomotor system can be affected by disturbances of the vestibular system in the inner ear, visuomotor complaints are common, but only rarely from injury to the visuomotor system in the brain stem.

Speech

After vision, speech is the next best understood function of the cerebral cortex. All representations of language — oral, written, and sign language — are first deciphered into meaningful language in Wernicke's area located in the left posterior temporal lobe. Expressions of language, whether they be in the form of speech, writings, or sign language, are initiated in Broca's area along the lateral side of the left frontal lobe. (Even in left handed people, speech is usually located in the left hemisphere.)

Disturbances of Wernicke's or Broca's area cause aphasia — mistakes in spelling or grammar. For example, the patient may say (or write) "streep" for street, or leave out prepositions, conjunctions, and other so-called helper words. Head trauma patients rarely suffer damage to the speech centers, probably because they are not subject to being thrust up against the interior of the skull.

Attention and Concentration

Less well understood functions of the brain are attention and concentration, memory, reasoning, judgment, thinking speed, and emotions. Obviously, the ability to focus attention was an important evolutionary advantage, and indeed, primitive areas of the brain (like the thalamus) play an important role in focusing and sustaining attention. What is less clear is the role played by more recent evolutionary additions to the brain — structures like the basal ganglia and the frontal, temporal, parietal, and occipital lobes.

Memory

The following are some general rules about memory loss. Recent memories are usually lost before established memories. Memories for facts are lost before memories for function (e.g., how to use a fork). Isolated inability to lay down new memories is usually due to medial temporal or perhaps thalamic damage. Thus, patients who cannot lay down new memories can still learn new motor skills, which are probably stored in the basal ganglia. Lesions of the superior frontal lobe tend to cause patients to forget when and where they first learned of the item being recalled. Lesions of the inferior frontal lobe (basal forebrain) alone rarely cause memory loss; the caudate nucleus of the basal ganglia must usually be involved, too.

Reasoning and Judgment

Reasoning is the ability to take a set of facts and arrive at the correct answer. Judgment is the ability to take a set of facts and arrive at the "best" answer when there is no correct one. Executive function — planning and strategizing for the future — is a good example of judgment where there is no correct answer, only a best one. Localization of reasoning and judgment is unclear.

Emotions

Emotions are another anatomically complex function. The limbic system plays the central role, but widespread areas of the cerebral cortex connected to the limbic system serve to modulate emotions. The limbic system begins in the temporal lobes and arches via the fornix into the inferior frontal regions and hypothalamus. The hypothalamus is the source for our involuntary responses to emotional situations — blushing, sweating, hair standing on end, pupillary dilation, rise in blood pressure, heart rate, and respiratory rate, diarrhea, bladder emptying, and erections.

Establishing a Diagnosis

Anatomic Differential Diagnosis

In general, neurologists arrive at a diagnosis in two logical steps. They first make an anatomic diagnosis — where is the problem — and then an etiologic diagnosis — now that I know where the problem is, what's causing it? The anatomic diagnosis begins during the history-taking. Listening to the patient's complaints, the neurologist begins to formulate anatomic possibilities to explain the symptoms. As more and more symptoms are elicited, the neurologist narrows the symptoms to a single anatomic spot. When more than one spot is considered, it is called an anatomic differential diagnosis.

Etiologic Differential Diagnosis

After (or while) establishing the anatomic differential diagnosis, the neurologist then considers all the possible etiologic insults for each spot in the anatomic differential diagnosis. This list of etiologic possibilities is called the etiologic differential diagnosis.

The neurologist tries to confirm the correct anatomic and etiologic diagnosis with the neurologic examination and neurologic tests like CAT scans, MRI, MRA (magnetic resonance angiography), SPECT scan, PET scan, EEG, BEAM (brain mapping), visual field testing, neuropsychologic testing, lumbar puncture, NCV (nerve conduction velocity) testing, EMG (electromyography), and various evoked studies involving vision, hearing, and touch.

Neurologic Tests

There are two types of neurologic tests: those that look at the structure of the brain and those that look at the function of the brain. The CAT scan and MRI look at the structure of the brain. The electroencephalogram (EEG), SPECT scan, PET scan, and evoked studies examine the function of the brain.

Anatomic Tests

MRI and CAT scan

The MRI and CAT scan slice the brain radiographically into slabs. The MRI does this with magnetic fields; the CAT scan uses x-rays. The MRI provides more detail than the CAT scan, but the CAT is superior to the MRI in detecting fresh blood in and around the brain. Being so sensitive, the MRI commonly detects brain damage in the normal population.

Physiologic Tests

MRA

MRA, or magnetic resonance angiography, is a means of visualizing the carotid and vertebral arterial systems in the neck and brain without having to inject contrast into the bloodstream. The resolution is not as good as with conventional arteriography, but the patient is spared the risks of catheterization and allergic reactions to the dye. (In conventional arteriography, a catheter is threaded from the femoral artery in the groin backward up the aorta into a carotid or vertebral artery in the neck, and then dye is injected up the catheter. As the dye flows into the brain, x-rays are taken of the cerebral vasculature.

An electroencephalogram monitors the brain's electrical activity by means of wires attached to the patient's scalp. These wires act like an antenna to record the brain's electrical activity. Normally, the resting brain emits signals at a frequency of 8 to 13 cycles per second (cps), called alpha activity, which is best seen in the occipital regions. Anything faster than 8-13cps is called beta activity. Slower rhythms include theta activity (6-7 cps) and delta activity (3-5 cps).

Theta and delta activity occur in the normal brain as the patient descends into sleep. If the patient is awake, any slowing of electrical activity in a focal area of the brain may indicate a lesion there. Similarly, widespread slowing indicates a widespread disturbance of brain function, often due to a bloodborne insult like low blood sugar, drug intoxication, liver failure, etc. "Spiking" discharges indicate an irritable area of cerebral cortex. If allowed to spread, the spikes can produce a seizure.

BEAM

Brain wave activity varies throughout the day depending on the state of alertness. Each area of the brain normally spends a characteristic amount of time in alpha, beta, theta, and delta activity. Brain mapping computers (BEAM) are now capable of creating a map of the brain's electrical activity depicting how long each area of the brain spends in each of the basic rhythms. By comparing the patient's map with that of a control population, it is possible to localize areas of focal slowing.

PET Scan

PET scanning (positron emission tomography) is based on the fact that the brain uses glucose for energy. By labeling a glucose molecule with a radioactive "tag," and then inhaling radioactive glucose and placing the patient's head under a large Geiger counter, one can identify abnormal areas of the brain that are underutilizing glucose. Because cyclotrons are needed to generate the radioactive gas, PET scanning is not widely available.

SPECT Scan

SPECT scanning (single photon emission computed tomography) is similar to PET scanning in that a radioactive chemical is given to the patient, but the radioactive chemical remains in the bloodstream and does not enter the brain. As a result, the SPECT scan maps the brain's vascular supply. Focal vascular defects on a SPECT scan are circumstantial evidence of brain damage. The advantage of a SPECT scan over a PET scan is its ready availability and relatively cheap cost.

Evoked Potentials

Evoked studies take advantage of the fact that each time a sensory system of the body — vision, hearing, touch — is stimulated, an electrical signal is generated in the brain. These electrical signals can be detected with electrical wires on the scalp. Thus, visual evoked recordings (VER) are recorded over the occipital lobes; brain stem auditory evoked recordings (BAER) over the temporal lobes; and somatosensory potentials (SSEP) over the parietal lobes.

Lumbar Puncture

A lumbar puncture (spinal tap) is used to analyze cerebrospinal fluid, the fluid in the ventricles and surrounding the brain and spinal cord. Because cerebrospinal fluid circulates from the brain down along the spinal cord, a lumbar puncture in the low back can detect abnormalities over two feet way in the brain. Typical abnormalities include elevated cerebrospinal fluid pressure, too many inflammatory white blood cells, elevated cerebrospinal fluid protein, abnormal proteins, antibodies to viruses, and the presence of various infectious agents.

Interpreting Neurologic Tests

Is the Test Abnormal?

In interpreting neurologic tests, one must first decide if the test is truly abnormal. For example, was the data correctly obtained and correctly interpreted? This problem arises with almost every study, and the only way to answer this question is to have the expert look at the raw data or actual images.

If the test were repeated on the same or, better yet, a different machine, would the result still be abnormal? Being so very sensitive, electrical tests (EEG, BEAM, VER, BAER, and SSEP) and radioactive scans (SPECT and PET) often produce a different result or even a normal result when repeated — hardly what you would expect from an area of fixed brain damage.

Was the test overread? An overread test is one in which the test result may be seen in both the normal and abnormal population, and the interpreter incorrectly chooses to place the patient among the abnormal population. This happens when a sizable segment of the control group scores in the abnormal range, or when the patient's test results are compared to a supernormal control group — for example, when a 70 year old's PET scan is compared to a group of 25 year olds. It is important, therefore, to make sure that the control, against which the patient was compared, was comparable to the patient.

The other reason an abnormal test result can be seen in both the normal and abnormal population is that the test is too sensitive and not specific enough. Sensitivity is the likelihood that a test will be abnormal — regardless of the cause of the brain malfunction. Specificity is the likelihood that an abnormal test result is due to a specific disease. In general, the more sensitive a test is, the less specific it is, because in making the test more sensitive, one begins to "pick up" more and more illnesses. In fact, tests can be so sensitive that nearly everyone scores abnormal because the test is picking up brain malfunction from anxiety over a family or employment problem, a bad night's sleep, mild depression, or side effect of medication. Ideally, a test should be made only sensitive enough to maximize its specificity.

What if the test is abnormal?

If the test is truly abnormal, one must then decide the following: Is the accident the actual cause of the abnormal test result? Is the abnormal area of brain indicated by the test capable of causing the patient's symptoms? Is the abnormal test result due to a pre-existing condition?

The Neurologic Evaluation

As the technology for CAT scans and MRI's has improved, so has their sensitivity and specificity. For EEG, brain mapping, evoked potentials, PET scanning, and SPECT scanning, however, sensitivity has improved without improvement in specificity. When tests become more sensitive without also becoming more specific, they are more likely to be abnormal because they detect more and more illnesses and more unusual states of normal physiology. Ironically, as a result of this technologic development, the independent neurologic exam has taken on greater significance. Abnormal neurologic test results have to be explained, and the answer usually lies in a thorough neurologic history and proper neurologic exam.

Simply put, there is no substitute for a face-to-face, hands-on evaluation of the patient. An experienced neurologist who understands the stress and inertia of a lawsuit can be of enormous help in sorting out the patient's complaints. It is not uncommon for patients to exaggerate their neurologic signs as a cry for help, or for health care providers to contribute unwittingly to the patient's neurologic problems. The correct diagnosis may have been missed, or proper treatment may have been overlooked. These situations can only be clarified by an independent neurologic exam.

The Neurologic History

One should reasonably expect a proper neurologic history to track the pattern and pace of a patient's complaints, including the things that make his symptoms worse and better, the effects of various treatments, and the effects his symptoms have had on his life. The neurologic history should note any past neurologic signs

- Objective neurologic abnormalities observable on neurologic exam
- And any past neurologic tests.

The Neurologic Exam

A complete neurologic exam includes an examination of five broad areas: the patient's mental status (his attentiveness, assertiveness, speed of thinking, speech, memory, judgment, affect, and insight); the cranial nerves (smell, visual acuity, visual fields, fundoscopy, eye movements, pupillary reaction, facial sensation and strength, hearing, articulation, and swallowing); the motor system (gait, atrophy, spasticity and rigidity, strength, coordination, involuntary movements, slowing of movements, and ataxia); the sensory system (vibration, proprioception, pain, temperature, double simultaneous stimulation); and the reflexes (biceps, triceps, knee, and ankle jerks, and Babinski signs).

Depending on the clinical problem, parts of the neurologic exam will obviously be expanded to look for additional neurologic signs, including signs of elaboration and inadequate effort.

CONCLUSION

There is no reason to be intimidated by a patient's impressive list of complaints or by the patient's abnormal neurologic tests, but in order to understand their significance, the patient must be referred to a neurologist experienced in dealing with patients involved in litigation, a neurologist who is unwilling to accept every complaint at face value. Many patients have convinced themselves, or been convinced by their health care providers, that they have suffered serious brain damage when, in fact, they are suffering from migraine or a psychological reaction fanned by the stress and inertia of the lawsuit. It is not uncommon for an entire family, including children, to be drawn into the patient's whirlpool of symptoms — symptoms which, if allowed to spiral out of control, will not stop at the resolution of litigation. These are complicated cases that require a neurologist capable of relating to the patient in a sympathetic and nurturing manner while maintaining a healthy distance from which he can gauge the significance of any abnormal neurologic tests.

SHELDON MARGULIES, M.D., J.D.

Located in Silver Springs, Maryland, Dr. Margulies is a Board Certified Neurologist. He received his medical degree from Stanford University and his law degree from the University of Baltimore School of Law. At the present time, Dr. Margulies maintains a private practice in neurology in Baltimore, Maryland where he is also on the faculty of Johns Hopkins University and University of Maryland. Dr. Margulies is a prolific writer having published textbooks in both medicine and law. His text, *Everyday Doctoring: A New Approach to the Logic and Reasoning of Neurology and Medicine,* is considered outstanding. He is awaiting publication of his text *Neuroanatomic Diagnoses in Everyday Practice.* He is the author of *Learning Law* outlining legal reasoning. Dr. Margulies has extensive experience with patients suffering head trauma, neuropsychological injuries, spinal cord injuries and toxic exposure. He has particular interests in medical malpractice and issues of causation.

9

THE PSYCHIATRIC EXAMINATION IN FORENSIC REHABILITATION

David E. Raskin, M.D.
Laurence R. Tancredi, M.D., J.D.

Traumatic brain injury is associated with a number of psychological and psychiatric problems. These are reflections of direct insult to the brain as well as reactions to decrease in function as a result of brain injury. The psychological problems include difficulties with cognitive functions such as deficits in attention, concentration and memory (Schwartz & McMillan, 1989) and changes in level of intelligence (Ewing-Cobbs et al., 1989) or in specific intellectual functions such as communication (Coelho et al., 1991) calculation abstraction (Rusonis, 1990), and insight and judgment. Recent studies have also shown alterations in the ability of injured parties to process information. Following traumatic head injuries, slowness in information processing is one of the main after effects (Tromp & Mulder, 1991). In addition personality changes may be seen in afflicted individuals (Michaud et al., 1993). These changes are usually characterized by either the development of new personality traits; for example, aggression in an individual who previously was mild and pleasant (Volavka et al., 1992), or an exaggeration of pre-existing personality traits. For example, a person who was previously compulsive and organized becomes more so as a way of dealing with the forgetfulness secondary to brain trauma. In addition to personality traits and aspects of cognitive function, there are psychiatric diagnoses which occur as a consequence of brain injury. These diagnoses cover a wide variety of DSM IV chapters. They include the development of organic mental disorders, the onset or exacerbation of psychotic disorders, the onset or exacerbation of affective disorders (Jorge et al., 1993), anxiety disorders, hysteria (Eames, 1992), somatoform disorders, and personality disorders. In essence then, any psychiatric disorder can occur as a consequence of brain dysfunction or be increased as a result of brain injury. It is important to note that a number of pre-existing factors will determine the kind and degree of psychiatric dysfunction seen after brain insult. Factors which need to be examined are a pre-existing history of one or more of the following: a psychiatric disorder, poor academic performance, problems in interpersonal relationships, and alcoholism and/or substance abuse. These interact with the severity of injury and specific part of the brain injured to produce post-injury effects. A recent study of depression in patients suffering acute traumatic brain injury supports the theory of multifactorial influences on the development of psychiatric disorders. This study (Fedoroff et al., 1992) involved 66 patients with closed head injuries. Of these 17 had major depression and two minor depressive symptoms — essentially 25% of patients suffering such injuries. The authors point out that this frequency of depression is similar to the frequency seen in other disorders such as cerebral vascular accidents. They also demonstrate that factors such as poor premorbid social functioning and the presence of previous psychiatric disorders is more frequent in these depressed patients. Finally, an important factor related to an increased incidence of depression is injury to critical parts of the brain such as the left dorsolateral frontal region, left basal ganglia, and to a lesser extent the parietal occipital region and right hemisphere.

This chapter will examine the following kinds of consequent problems: 1) Axis I disorders and 2) personality disorders as a consequence of brain injury. It will also review methods of diagnosis of the psychiatric complications of traumatic brain injury which are available for forensic examination.

Psychiatric Disturbances

Axis I Disorders

As previously stated, Axis I disorders can be viewed as a consequence of direct insult to the brain and/or a reaction to a decline in function as a result of injury to the brain. It is clear from the studies of Robinson and others that certain areas of the brain are more susceptible to injury and can produce fairly specific psychiatric symptoms.

Depression is a common consequence of brain trauma and can be conceptualized as either a direct reflection of underlying brain dysfunction or a reaction to it. In order to make this distinction, the time of onset is helpful. The depression which occurs as a consequence of brain injury looks no different from a depression without brain injury. However, because of the possibility of interference with concentration and memory as a direct result of brain injury, it is often difficult to determine whether these symptoms reflect the symptoms of depression or the symptoms of brain trauma. Basically, the best way to make this distinction is through the use of antidepressants which should treat concentration and memory problems as a result of depression but be ineffective in concentration and memory problems which are a direct reflection of brain injury.

Depressive disorders secondary to brain injury have a whole variety of symptoms and signs consistent with non-injury depressed disorders. Treatment is very much the same, that is, the use of antidepressants. However, there may be dose differences because of pharmacodynamic considerations. People with brain injury are often more sensitive to medications and will respond to lower doses and will often develop side effects at doses lower than usually seen.

Another syndrome now well described in the literature is post-traumatic mania. There are a group of patients who develop manic syndromes, once again, not at all phenomenologically different from primary mania as a result of head injury. Agitation and maladaptive behavior may also be seen in brain injured patients unrelated to the presence of mania or depression. Antianxiety drugs may be useful in treating this condition. There has been some success with the use of low-dose buspirone (Ratey et al., 1992). Another common phenomenon of vascular or traumatic brain injury is emotional lability. This may also not be associated with either depression or manic features. However, it is an embarrassing condition for the sufferer who may not be able to exert any control over its manifestations. Presently, there appears to be no satisfactory method of treatment for this condition (Allman, 1992). However, research using fluoxetine, a relatively new antidepressant which focuses on serotonergic action, seems promising. In one study involving six cases of emotional lability secondary to brain injury (five from strokes and one from traumatic brain injury), all of the patients showed significant improvement within one week of using fluoxetine (Sloan et al., 1992).

Besides affective disorders we see the presence of schizophrenic disorders sometimes as a consequence of direct injury to the brain. These schizophrenic disorders can be of any variety although they are often of a paranoid type, and they are best treated with the use of antipsychotic medications. Once again, these medications need to be utilized in appropriate dosage and consideration of side effects is paramount.

Generalized anxiety disorder and panic disorder are another set of diagnoses which are fairly common after traumatic brain injury. One type of anxiety disorder, catastrophic anxiety, is often seen when people with traumatic brain injury are questioned about areas of deficit. They become explosively angry and/or anxious, and the sensitive interviewer needs to keep this in mind when working with such patients.

Personality Disorders as a Consequence of Injury

Personality disorders are a frequent consequence of traumatic brain injury. As stated previously, these may be reflective of new personality traits. Prominent among these are the traits of irritability and anger of an explosive kind. These effects can be set off as stated in the previous paragraph. As explosive as these effects are, they can be diminished by a calm redirection of the patient during the interview.

Suspiciousness is another trait which can be found subsequent to injury. Lability of affect with people crying easily, laughing inappropriately, and being viewed as moody by their families is another trait. In people with frontal lobe syndrome, impaired social judgment, labile affect, inappropriate behavior, and poor hygiene are all found. The treatment of the psychiatric sequelae of traumatic brain injury is quite similar to the treatment of primary psychiatric disorder. These are some issues which need to be attended to; however, it is important that the treatment be conducted in an environment which is conducive to improvement. Such an environment for post-traumatic patients is one in which stress, extreme affects, and change of environment are kept to a minimum. A simple, consistent, organized, rational environment will yield better results than one in which there are multiple unexpected changes; an environment in which people are calm and collected rather than frustrated and angry will produce better results. It may require working with the patient's average expected environment, that is, with family, group home or hospital, in order to provide such an environment within which antidepressants or antipsychotic medicine can be prescribed.

In addition to the treatment of primary psychiatric disorders, there are very specific treatments for the aggressive disorders seen after traumatic brain injury. These treatments include the use of Lithium, Carbamazepine, beta blockers, and occasionally antipsychotics to control post-traumatic aggression. It is hard to find good data on percentage improvement of these patients, particularly because little time is spent on attempting to control the environment in which medications are being used. This lack of environmental control causes great variance in treatment response. Dosages, as stated previously, need to be at lower levels than in the ordinary primary psychiatric patient, and attention needs to be paid to side effect issues.

Forensic Issues and Diagnostic Methods

The forensic psychiatrist is often asked to intervene in cases of post-traumatic psychiatric disorder. It is important that clear thinking and careful distinctions be made in these cases.

The problem case is one in which a litigant, who denies pre-existing problems, claims that a mild head injury, often without loss of consciousness or amnesia, has lead to serious memory difficulties. Many of these cases represent two underlying problems. In one, the legal environment, including physicians as well as attorneys, focus the patient on their memories to the extent that patients, particularly those with obsessional personality traits, begin to identify normal variances in memory, become anxious about these, catalogue them, worry about them, and describe them as post-injury memory problems. The second underlying problem for memory difficulties is the litigant who is exaggerating or dissembling memory difficulties. In the paradigm cases, for both of these claimants, there is a marked distinction between their subjective complaints and their objective performance in the office when they are unaware that their memory is being examined. These same claimants, when given specific testing of a psychological or neuropsychological kind, often perform poorly, yet when giving a history of doctors, procedures, and dates of injury and treatment are able to do this in a compelling way. It is also not uncommon to find in the group of claimants who either have ruminations about memory or are dissembling about memory that their activities of daily living are inconsistent with a memory problem. These are often claimants who are able to take care of children, including the complicated tasks of feeding on schedule, getting them to various places, and controlling their behavior. They are often claimants who are able to drive in complicated cities without problem.

It is important to note that although we see a variety of psychiatric problems in true post-traumatic injury, most often of a personality change kind in the ruminating obsessional patient and the dissembling patient, it is often memory which is focused upon. They rarely complain of personality problems except for increases in irritability.

In order to assess and distinguish the legitimate cases of post-injury psychiatric disorder, i.e., depression, psychosis, anxiety disorder or personality disorder, from the cases of obsessional focusing or dissembling, a careful forensic psychiatric exam needs to be performed. This includes 1) examining medical records, 2) performing a detailed and systematic forensic clinical evaluation, and 3) conducting focused psychological testing.

A. Medical Records

Medical records are critical to determine whether or not the injury is the problem or there are pre-existing issues. Medical records of importance include physicians' records which will often document the use of drugs and alcohol which affect cognitive function, school records which often document the presence of poor academic performance and hyperactivity, military records which often document interpersonal difficulties, and employment records which will often document a variety of interpersonal and cognitive difficulties. Without a systematic record review, it is truly impossible to determine whether post-traumatic head injury patients are experiencing true responses to trauma or other forces are operative.

B. The Clinical Evaluation

The clinical evaluation of these individuals should utilize an indirect, non-question and answer approach in order to assess baseline performance. A psychiatric exam which attends to the claimant's behavior and leads to a mental status is more appropriate than focused questioning. In the indirect exam, one often encounters a discrepancy between subjective and objective performance.

Many new diagnostic technologies have been found useful in evaluating the presence and extent of injury. Computerized Axial Tomography (CT) scans have been used to establish the extent of structural changes in the brain following a traumatic injury. Scans can establish the amount of cerebral damages once the acute changes in the brain have resolved. These findings have been correlated with neuropsychological status of the patient. A recent study (Reider-Groswasser et al., 1993) demonstrates the relationship of late CT findings to psychological sequelae and to potential vocational rehabilitation. This study focused primarily on patients receiving severe blunt brain trauma. It involved 32 men who received severe trauma but had been healthy in the premorbid state. The researchers found a high correlation between the width of the third ventricle and outcomes in terms of return of cognitive abilities and vocational rehabilitation. It is hypothesized that the width of the third ventricle is a useful index of diffuse brain trauma.

In addition to CT scans, other diagnostic tools such as quantitative electroencephalography (QEEG) and cerebral blood flow measurements are useful in assessing the extent of brain damage. All of these measures focus on the correlation of structural changes with cognitive and behavioral sequelae and have been used to correlate the effects of premorbid conditions (such as substance abuse, psychiatric disorders etc.) on the severity of outcomes following head trauma (Ronty et al., 1993).

With the development of technologies such as magnetic resonance imaging (MRI), single photon emission computerized tomography (SPECT) and more recently positron emission tomography (PET) there has been a major advance in the diagnostic capacity of the forensic psychiatrist. These technologies not only enhance the accuracy and precision of demonstrating structural changes brought on by injuries, but they also allow for the direct biological assessment of functional impairment (Volkow & Tancredi, 1986). MRI has been used for some time as a complementary diagnostic measure to CT scans. CT scans seem most useful in evaluating initially the acutely unstable patient. However, MRI offers the opportunity of identifying many lesions (Yokota et al., 1991) such as small subdural hematomas, cortical contusions, and diffuse axonal injuries which are not picked up by CT examination (Sklar et al., 1992). In addition to being clinically useful in assessing vascular abnormalities, MRI seems superior to CT in assessing pediatric trauma (Sklar et al., 1992).

In some studies SPECT has been shown to be superior to CT and MRI in demonstrating focal cerebral lesions (Newton et al., 1992). Both SPECT and PET have the capacity of showing functional changes in the brain. SPECT is a much less costly instrument than PET for use in clinical diagnosis; however, in its current development it is not as specific and precise an instrument (Volkow & Tancredi, 1992). With the use of radio-labeled glucose it is possible to show changes in metabolism in areas of the brain where structural lesions may not be apparent by either CT Scan or MRI. PET has been used for some time as a research tool in assessing brain dysfunction (Volkow & Tancredi, 1992). PET studies have been useful in demonstrating functional changes associated with a wide variety of conditions including violent behavior associated with brain trauma (Volkow & Tancredi, 1987). In recent years MRI has also been developed to play an increasing role in examining functional processes in the brain (Buckley et al., 1993). It is promising to be an important tool in evaluating functional differences in parts of the brain, differences which would not be apparent in an examination of structural changes. In some cases MRI is being shown to be complementary to PET. It has the advantage over PET and SPECT of not requiring the introduction intravenously of a radioactive material.

C. Psychological Testing

There are a variety of psychological tests which can be used to help clarify whether or not post-injury problems are, in fact, legitimate. Any claimant can perform poorly on psychological testing because of poor motivation related to a number of causes. In addition to its use as a method for profiling patients suffering from emotional disturbances following head trauma (Leininger et al., 1991), the Minnesota Multiphasic Personality Inventory (MMPI) allows for an examination of motivation and performance and helps determine whether or not the person is validly performing the test (Gass & Russell, 1991). In addition, there are now other tests for assessment brain injured patients such as the Millon Clinical Multiaxial Inventory (MCMI) which is used to assess personality changes following head injuries (Tuokko et al., 1991), the Warrington Recognition Memory Test which is used to detect memory impairment (Millis & Dijkers, 1993) and several tests such as the Rey Memory Test which can identify dissembling behavior.

Conclusion

This discussion has reviewed the major psychiatric conditions frequently associated with traumatic brain injury. The most important conditions involve major personality and behavioral disorders, cognitive and memory impairments and the development of serious psychiatric conditions, particularly the affective disorders. The etiology of these conditions in any one patient is most likely to be more complex than exposure to brain trauma alone. Though in fact the brain trauma may serve as the most critical precipitating event and therefore must be carefully evaluated.

Through the use of a careful examination of records, a clever, indirect examination, the application of appropriate biological diagnostic measures such as the use of new technologies (SPECT, PET, MRI) and psychological testing, the forensic psychiatrist is fortified in his ability to properly diagnose a patient's condition. Such an evaluation will enable him to distinguish between legitimate psychiatric problems that are a response to traumatic brain injury from the psychiatric problems which appear to be related to other factors. If, however, the exam is naively performed without records or psychological testing and is based on more or less question and answer, a distorted view of causality and function will be obtained.

References

Allman, P. (1992). Drug treatment of emotionalism following brain damage. *Journal of The Royal Society of Medicine, 85(7),* 423-424.

Buckley, P., Stack, J.P., Madigan C., et al, (1993). Magnetic resonance imaging of schizophrenia-like psychoses associated with cerebral trauma: Clinicopathological correlates. *American Journal of Psychiatry, 150(1),* 146-148.

Coelho, C.A., Liles, B.Z. & Duffy, R.J. (1991). Discourse analyses with closed head injured adults: Evidence for differing patterns of deficits. *Archives of Physical Medicine and Rehabilitation, 72(7),* 465-468.

Eames, P. (1992). Hysteria following brain injury. *Journal of Neurology, Neurosurgery and Psychiatry, 55(11),* 1046-1053.

Ewing-Cobbs, L., Miner, M.D., Fletcher, J.D., et al, (1989). Intellectual, motor, and language sequelae following closed head injury in infants and preschoolers. *Journal of Pediatric Psychology, 14(4),* 531-547.

Fedoroff, J.P., Starkstein, S.E., Forrester, A.W., et al, (1992). Depression in patients with acute traumatic brain injury. *American Journal of Psychiatry, 149(7),* 918-921.

Gass, C.S. & Russell, E.W. (1991). MMPI profiles of closed head trauma patients: Impact of neurologic complaints. *Journal of Clinical Psychology, 47(2),* 253-260.

Jorge, R.E., Robinson, R.G., Arndt, S.V., et al, (1993). Comparison between acute- and delayed-onset depression following traumatic brain injury. *Journal of Neuropsychiatry and Clinical Neurosciences,* 5(1) 43-49.

Leininger, B.E., Dreutzer, J.D., Hill, M.R. (1991). Comparison of minor and severe head injury emotional sequelae using the MMPI. *Brain Injury, 5(2),* 199-205.

Michaud, L.T., Rivara, F.P., Jaffe, K.M., et al, (1993). Traumatic brain injury as a risk factor for behavioral disorders in children. *Archives of Physical Medicine and Rehabilitation, 74(4),* 368-375.

Millis, S.R. & Dijkers, M. (1993). Use of the recognition memory test in traumatic brain injury: Preliminary findings. *Brain Injury, 7(1),* 53-58.

Newton, M.R., Greenwood, R.J., Britton, K.E., et al, (1992). A study comparing SPECT with CT and MRI after closed head injury. *Journal of Neurology, Neurosurgery and Psychiatry, 55(2)*, 92-94.

Ratey, J.J., Leveroni, C.L., Miller, A.C., et al, (1992). Low-dose buspirone to treat agitation and maladaptive behavior in brain-injured patients: Two case reports. *Journal of Clinical Psychopharmacology, 12(5)*, 362-364.

Reider-Groswasser, I., Cohen, M., Costeff, H. (1993). Late CT findings in brain trauma: Relationship to cognitive and behavioral sequelae and to vocational outcome. *American Journal of Roentgennology, 160(1)*, 147-152.

Ronty, H., Ahonen, A., Tolonen, U., et al, (1993). Cerebral trauma and alcohol abuse. *European Journal of Clinical Investigation, 23(3)*, 182-187.

Rusonis, E.S. (1990). Adolescents with closed head injury: Neuropsychological consequences. *Medical Clinics of North America, 74(5)*, 1311-1319.

Schwartz, A. F., & McMillan, T.M. (1989). Assessment of everyday memory after severe head injury. *Cortex, 24(4)*, 665-671.

Sklar, E.M., Quencer, R.M., Bowen, B.C., et al, (1992). Magnetic resonance applications in cerebral injury. *Radiologic Clinics of North America, 30(2)*, 353-366.

Sloan, R.L., Brown, K.W., Pentland, B. (1992). Fluoxetine as a treatment for emotional lability after brain injury. *Brain Injury, 6(4)*, 315-319.

Tromp, E., Mulder, T. (1991). Slowness of information processing after traumatic head injury. *Journal of Clinical and Experimental Neuropsychology, 13(6)*, 821-830.

Tuokko, H., Vernon-Wilkinson, R., Robinson, E. (1991). The use of the MCMI in the personality assessment of head-injury adults. *Brain Injury, 5(3)*, 287-293.

Volavka, J., Martell, D., Convit, A. (1992). Psychobiology of the violent offender. *Journal of Forensic Sciences, 37(1)*, 237-251.

Volkow, N. & Tancredi, L. (1986). Positron emission tomography: A technology assessment. *International Journal of Technology Assessment in Health Care, 2*, 577-594.

Volkow, N. & Tancredi, L. (1987). Neural substrates of violent behavior: A preliminary study with positron emission tomography. *British Journal of Psychiatry, 151*, 668-673.

Volkow, N. & Tancredi, L. (1992). Current and future applications of SPECT in clinical psychiatry. *Journal of Clinical Psychiatry, 53* (11 suppl), 26-28.

Yokota, H., Kurakowa, A., Otsuka, T., et al, (1991). Significance of magnetic resonance imaging in acute head injury. *Journal of Trauma, 31(3)*, 351-357

David E. Raskin, M.D.

Located in Wilmington, Delaware, Dr. Raskin is a Clinical Professor in the Department of Psychology and Human Behavior at Jefferson Medical College of Philadelphia, Pennsylvania. He is also a surveyor and teacher for the Joint Commission for Accreditation of Health Care Organizations and a psychiatric consultant for the correctional facilities in Delaware. Dr. Raskin is Board certified in Psychiatry by the American Board of Psychiatry and Neurology and Board Certified in Forensic Psychiatry by the American Board of Forensic Psychiatry. He is also a Diplomate of the American Board of Quality Assurance and Utilization Review Physicians. Dr. Raskin has been licensed in numerous states, including California, Connecticut, District of Columbia, Illinois, Washington, Virginia, Delaware, Pennsylvania, and Maryland. He is currently licensed in Maryland, Delaware, and Pennsylvania, and has offices in those states. Dr. Raskin has presented on numerous occasions at national association meetings, including the American Academy of Clinical Psychiatrists, the National Council on Aging, and the American Academy of Psychiatry and the Law. Dr. Raskin has 65 publications regarding psychiatry, treatment, and diagnostic issues.

Laurence R. Tancredi, M.D., J.D.

Laurence R. Tancredi, M.D., J.D. is a physician-lawyer with board certification in psychiatry. He is currently in private practice in New York City. He previously was the Kraft Eidman Professor of Medicine and the Law, and Professor of Psychiatry at the University of Texas Health Science Center in Houston. He has authored many articles for medical, psychiatric, and legal journals, and has authored or co-authored several books, including a textbook of clinical psychiatry *Clinical Psychiatric Medicine* and a handbook of psychiatric emergencies. He has participated on national and international committees, presented papers at professional and scientific meetings and is a member of several professional organizations, including the American Psychiatric Association, the American Academy of Psychiatry and Law, the American Society of Law and Medicine, and the International Academy of Psychiatry and Law. Dr. Tancredi is a graduate of the University of Pennsylvania School of Medicine and the Yale School of Law. He currently engages in psychiatric resident supervision, medical research and forensic psychiatry practice.

10

THE NEUROPSYCHOLOGICAL EVALUATION IN FORENSIC REHABILITATION

Harold H. Smith, Ph.D., ABPP

Hundreds of thousands of individuals are injured yearly in motor vehicle accidents or falls (rapid accelerative or decelerative forces), during assault (when the head is stationary), and are acutely and chronically exposed to a variety of industrial toxins. Many of these individuals require intensive efforts to save their lives, and after treatment for the acute phase of their injury may receive additional treatment in a rehabilitation facility and receive evaluation and treatment from several professional disciplines. Some individuals may receive evaluation and treatment in a structured hospital based program, where physical speech difficulties may also be attended. Many others who have been subjected to a mild or moderate injury may receive various evaluations and treatment approaches as outpatients. Many will initiate lawsuits.

Persons having more severe injuries, and particularly those for whom neurodiagnostic procedures, such as computer axial tomography or magnetic resonance imaging have provided objective evidence of damage to the brain parenchyma, vessels, or coverings, may be readily understood when they voice complaints about their diminished emotional control or cognitive functions. Often they have visible evidence of the trauma which they survived, or manifest speech and language deficits which immediately identify them as having had a disruption in brain functioning. To understand how higher level cognitive abilities have been affected, a neuropsychological examination is conducted to document the injured person's level of functioning, establish treatment approaches, measure subsequent improvement or decline in functioning, provide prognosis including needs for future psychotherapy or other intervention, and guide decisions regarding everyday activities and employment. For a complete discussion of neuropsychological examination as it relates to rehabilitation procedures, the reader is referred to Goldstein & Ruthven (1983), Prigatano, Fordyce, Zainer, Roueche, Pepping & Wood (1986), and Ellis & Christensen (1989).

When neurodiagnostic studies are negative and the patient continues to complain of impaired cognitive functioning, a neuropsychological examination often is the next effort made to clarify the nature of the person's difficulties. Dacey, Vollmer & Kikmen (1993) have concluded that neuropsychological changes after mild head injury are time limited, particularly in young healthy persons having an uncomplicated mild head injury. Genuine cognitive deficits, emotional responses to injury and fear of injury to the "organ of the mind", as well as malingering, symptom magnification, and conversion disorder must be assessed against the background of the nature of the injury (see Gennarelli, 1993).

Within the health care setting a neuropsychological examination is usually requested by a physician, such as a neurologist or psychiatrist, or may be part of a comprehensive evaluation within a rehabilitation facility. Increasingly plaintiff's attorneys are also requesting neuropsychological examinations of their clients as they recognize that this type of examination provides much more information regarding the functions of the brain which can be affected by trauma or toxic exposure. Defense counsel usually respond with an independent neuropsychological examination, and when there is lack of agreement the battle is usually between the testimony of neuropsychologist versus neuropsychologist or physician. The claims representative also has to become familiar with neuropsychological terms and concepts in order to be able to best evaluate claims of brain damage.

The Examination

The nature of a neuropsychological examination varies tremendously. Occasionally a psychologist or psychiatrist may have a patient draw nine geometric designs and comment on whether there is evidence for "organicity". This unitary concept of brain damage is, however, usually regarded as an unacceptable simplification of impaired brain functioning. Some psychologists give several "neuropsychological screening tests" and make a decision about the presence or absence of cerebral dysfunction. Most neuropsychologists, however, would be expected to administer a variety of exclusive neuropsychological assessment procedures to sample different domains of brain functioning. This is recommended because a comprehensive neuropsychological examination is more sensitive to cerebral dysfunction than traditional psychological procedures (Goldstein, Deysach, & Kleinknecht, 1973), neurological examination, electroencephalogram, and the now obsolete pneumoencephalogram, and it compares well with the hit rates for computer axial tomography (Tsushima & Wedding, 1979) and magnetic resonance imaging. There is, however, no national standard for what comprises a "neuropsychological battery", but the Halstead-Reitan Neuropsychological Test Battery, the Luria Neuropsychological Test Battery, and the Boston approach to neuropsychological testing, as well as an "eclectic" approach are most often used.

The Examiner

Persons of diverse backgrounds administer these neuropsychological tests. The practice of psychology, or the protection of the title, "psychologist", is regulated by a generic license. Thus, anyone licensed as a psychologist could refer to himself as being a "neuropsychologist" because that title is not regulated. Nonetheless, ethical conduct would require that a person who claims neuropsychology as an area of practice would possess the requisite education, training, and experience to offer such services. Older psychologists, particularly those trained in clinical psychology, most likely received their training in this practice area from attendance at postdoctoral workshops, independent study, and occasionally, supervised interpretation of the test instruments. Today, one can obtain a doctoral degree in neuropsychology, or obtain mastery of this practice area through completion of postdoctoral residency training programs. Mastery of the subject area of neuropsychology is also recognized through certification by the American Board of Professional Psychology and the American Board of Professional Neuropsychology.

Neuropsychological examinations are conducted by persons having different training and experience backgrounds, and differ in their diagnostic abilities. From my review of reports, persons holding the Doctor of Philosophy (Ph.D.) degree as well as the Doctor of Psychology (Psy. D.) degree, with their training focus having been in the areas of clinical, counseling, experimental, physiological or school psychology provide this clinical service. The neuropsychological examination, particularly in forensic cases, should be conducted by the professional having the greatest education, training, and experience in this specialty field.

Some examinations, however, are conducted by persons who do not have a degree in psychology, but were licensed as psychologists because their training was primarily "psychological in nature". Some neuropsychological examinations are conducted by persons holding a Masters degree, most often in those jurisdictions which license psychologists at the master's degree level. Sometimes neuropsychological examinations are conducted by recent doctoral degree recipients who are completing a period of supervised practice in order to meet requirements for licensure. They collect the test data, and sometimes write or contribute to a report. In some university settings graduate students conduct the examinations, and sometimes several students or psychology residents will conduct different parts of an examination of the same patient. When an examination is conducted as part of the training of a psychologist there exists considerable opportunity for error, as has been noted by Slate, Jones and Murray (1991) and Moon,

Blakey, Gorsuch and Fantuzzo (1991).

Not uncommonly, a psychiatrist may hire a technician to conduct neuropsychological examinations. The qualifications of the technician varies considerably, ranging from masters level in psychology or social work, to high school graduate who also serves as secretary/receptionist. Plaintiff's counsel may occasionally be in a position to select the professional to conduct the neuropsychological examination, and as a general rule, defense counsel has considerable choice of who to select. Careful scrutiny should be given to the psychologist's education, training, and experience. It is not enough to accept an "expert" in neuropsychology an individual who has met only the basic requirements for licensure.

Post Concussion Syndrome

In personal injury cases a neuropsychological examination is recommended whenever the client has symptoms related to central nervous system functioning and has been exposed to trauma or toxic exposure. The presence of post concussion syndrome, a condition in which loss of consciousness is not necessary for its signs and symptoms to develop (Evans, 1992), would be a threshold condition for conducting a detailed examination. The most common elements of this syndrome include headaches, dizziness, fatigue, irritability, anxiety, insomnia, diminished concentration and memory, as well as heightened sensitivity to noise. Various other symptoms may be reported as well, including vertigo, tinnitus, diminished hearing, blurred vision or double vision as well as hypersensitivity to light, altered perceptions of taste and smell, slowed reaction time and information processing speed, decreases in appetite and sexual interest, as well as personality changes. The validity of the post concussion syndrome continues to be disputed, in part because many of its components occur with a high base rate in the normal population, and because of bias on the part of the victim (Mittenberg, DiGiulio, Perrin, & Bass,1992). As the research designs improve in studies of patients having these complaints, and diagnostic procedures become more sensitive, we can expect to arrive at a better understanding of the basis of this syndrome.

Thompson (1965) noted that early post concussion syndrome objective findings would include "changes in the size and shape of the pupils, disturbances of ocular convergence, difficulty in coordination and balance, nystagmus, dilation of the retinal vessels, postural defects, defective associative moments, and sometimes alteration of the deep reflexes and the transient presence of pathological reflexes (p.1016)." He also reported a variety of subjective symptoms that include headache, dizziness, nervous tension, irritability, insomnia, confusion, memory problems, and difficulties with concentration and emotional stability.

Many injured persons do not develop post concussion syndrome, but present with specific cognitive complaints, particularly impaired memory. Neuropsychological impairments may be related to focal and/or diffuse injuries; however, localization of deficits is often difficult because many neuropsychological tests are sensitive to brain injury regardless of localization of damage.

Post Traumatic Stress Disorder

Sometimes the post-concussion syndrome is confused with the post-traumatic stress disorder (PTSD). Litz and Keane (1989) noted that some of the key defining characteristics of PTSD included symptoms that affect perceptual, attentional, and memory processes; however, Dalton, Pederson, and Ryan (1989) suggested that Vietnam veteran PTSD patients had only minor deviations from normative samples on intelligence and several neuropsychological tests (no control group was used). McCaffrey, Hickling, and Marrazo (1989) have cautioned that the assessment strategies and diagnostic decision rules developed for use with Vietnam veterans have limited application to PTSD symptoms in the civilian population. In the general population, symptoms of PTSD may precede a cause of litigation, and include such experiences as a spouse's affair, being poisoned, and having a miscarriage (Helzer, Robins & McEvoy, 1987). It can be assumed that some civil cases may include factitious claims of PTSD based on the findings of

Sparr and Pankratz (1983) and Lynn and Belza (1984), and extrapolating from Perconte and Goreczny (1990) diagnostic tests may not clearly differentiate the malingerer. Finally, Platt and Husband (1985) and Raifman (1983) have addressed various forensic issues related to the PTSD diagnosis, which should be reviewed by persons expecting to defend that diagnosis in court.

Premorbid Functioning

Intelligence test scores are robust and as measures of "crystallized" and overlearned abilities, are not likely to be altered by trauma unless it is severe, and even then improvement is expected as the patient recovers. Some examiners have claimed that their patient has undergone a decline in his level of intellect based upon the scatter or variation among subtest scaled scores. For example, examiners have been known to use the one or two highest scores as an indicator of premorbid intellect, and such a procedure is not valid, as has been thoroughly reviewed by Matarazzo (1990). In conjunction with other demographic and test data, however, certain subtests of intelligence scales may allow one to make an estimate of the level of functioning prior to the trauma or exposure. Intelligence tests alone are insufficient for making a determination about the existence of cognitive deficit due to trauma. They do, however, provide the background for interpretation of performances on "fluid" abilities.

A patient's level of premorbid functioning may also be estimated through the use of historical records (academic, military, employment, or prior examinations) and with the use of tests of academic achievement, such as the Wide Range Achievement Test (in which the patient pronounces words, writes the spelling of words, and figures math problems and records their answers) or the Peabody Individual Achievement Test (in which the patient gives an oral multiple choice response to math, spelling, reading recognition and general information items, and pronunciation) , or the use of the National Adult Reading Test (the patient pronounces words with irregular spelling). Periodically, new achievement tests are introduced which generally tap the same type of abilities. With sufficient historical, intellectual, and achievement test data reasonable estimates of premorbid functioning may be made.

Intellectual Examination

The interpretation of neuropsychological test results is dependent upon several demographic variables, including level of intellect, age, educational attainment, and gender, as well as history of alcohol use and, coexisting physical ailments unrelated to the trauma, or toxic exposure. Adult intelligence is usually measured using the Wechsler Adult Intelligence Scale-Revised (WAIS-R) or the earlier edition (WAIS), although the condition of the patient may require other instruments, such as the Peabody Picture Vocabulary Test or Raven Progressive Matrices. Children's intelligence is assessed using the Wechsler Intelligence Scale for Children-III (WISC-III) or the earlier edition (WISC-R, or the Stanford Binet Intelligence Scale. Younger children may have intelligence assessed using the Wechsler Preschool and Primary Scale of Intelligence (WPPSI). Scaled scores on the Wechsler Scales are derived according to age, and additional age corrected norms allow direct comparison of scores to others in a specific age group. Additional norms are available for persons beyond age 74 (Ivnik, Malec, Smith, Tangalos, Petersen, Kokmen & Kurland, 1992) Examiners who fail to adhere to standardized administration procedures and do not record verbatim the patient's responses diminish the value of their findings because the raw data upon which they base their conclusions are not available for the scrutiny of others.

Neuropsychological Tests

Neuropsychological tests have been described in several texts (Reitan & Davison, 1974; Lezak, 1983; Hartman, 1988; Spreen & Strauss, 1991, Reitan & Wolfson, 1992) and a summary of reliability and validity studies has been provided by Franzen (1989). Recently Heaton, Grant, and Matthews (1991) presented comprehensive norms for an expanded Halstead-Reitan Battery that included demographic corrections for age, educational attainment, and gender. Research journals frequently publish norms for various tests, and these as well must be considered when interpreting an individual set of scores.

Regardless of the neuropsychological testing approach which is used, it is important to survey the various functions of the brain when a patient is likely to be involved in litigation. A more focused examination may be more appropriate when an individual has a discrete lesion with specific impairments, such as aphasia, and the focus is to establish a rehabilitation program.

An examination of various aspects of attention (Mirsky, 1987, Mirsky, Anthony, Duncan, Ahearn & Kellam, 1991, Shum, McFarland & Bain, 1990) and speed of information processing (Johnson, Roethig-Johnson & Middleton, 1988, Brittain, LaMarche, Reeder, Roth & Boll, 1991) is important even though the patient is alert and oriented. These various tests of attention and information processing measure one's abilities to focus attention and execute behavior, encode information, sustain attention (vigilance), shift attention, and respond rapidly to rapidly presented test stimuli. These basic mental processes may be affected by concussion and brain damage, and have significance for the social and employment opportunities of injured persons.

Impairments in memory functioning are some of the most frequent complaints of individuals who have sustained a head injury (Levin, Benton & Grossman, 1982) or who have had toxic exposure (Miller & Eckerman, 1986). In cases of traumatic brain injury the patient may have total amnesia for events immediately prior to the trauma (retrograde amnesia); however, as their condition improves the period of amnesia diminishes to the point that memory loss may exist only for a few seconds prior to trauma. Amnesia may also exist for the a period of time during recovery from an injury (post-traumatic amnesia) and may extend from moments to several weeks. This amnesia may exist even though the patient may have been conscious and communicating with caretakers or family. Sometimes individuals complain of loss of remote memories, which may be restored, but the most common complaint involves difficulty in the call of ongoing everyday activities and experiences. It is this latter short term memory difficulty which poses the most problems for traumatically brain injured persons.

There are various types of memory tests, and two of the better known standardized ones are the Wechsler Memory Scale-Revised (WMS-R) and the California Verbal Learning Test (CVLT). Each of these instruments has been the focus of continuing validity and reliability studies and much has been learned about the memory functioning of persons having various disorders. Separate indices may be calculated from scores on the WMS-R, including visual and verbal memory, from which a general memory index is derived, and measures of attention/concentration and delayed recall. Norms for persons older than age 74 have been provided by Ivnic, Malec, Tangalos, Petersen, Kokmen and Kurland (1992).

The CVLT reflects learning performance across five trials as the patient is asked to learn sixteen words which are orally presented. Memory and learning measures include free recall, meaning recall of the words in any order, over the five trials and after an interference list has been introduced, and cued recall, meaning that a general category cue is offered to assist recall. After a twenty minute delay, during which another activity is undertaken to prevent active rehearsal of the words, additional free and cued recall measures are taken, as well as a recognition measure. The recognition memory measure requires the patient to identify the original list items which are presented with distractor items from the interference list and items never presented. These measures provide much useful information regarding the strategies a person uses to organize and retain information, and quantifies this data for comparison with normative and patient groups (Crosson, Novack, Trenerry & Craig, 1988).

There exists a variety of other memory tests; however, the examiner should carefully attend to how well the test has withstood critical review. Readers of results from memory tests should also be aware that even the better memory tests require considerable attention on the part of the examiner to meet standardized testing procedures. Further, some psychologists have commented on the likely anatomical site of a lesion causing a memory dysfunction, usually the medial aspect of the temporal lobes and/or the hyppocampal formation. The level of certainty with which such statements are made could be considered to be relatively low in view of the fact that memory functioning may require input from multiple brain sites.

One of the hallmarks of brain damage, particularly the frontal lobes, is impaired ability to abstract (Goldstein & Scheerer, 1941). Higher level reasoning and conceptual ability is often measured by means of the Category Test, considered by many to be the most sensitive of the Halstead-Reitan measures to cerebral dysfunction. The Trail Making Test-Part B measures not only attention, but also aspects of abstraction. Other measures of abstract reasoning, problem solving, and conceptual flexibility include the Wisconsin Card Sorting Test, Shipley Institute of Living Scale, and Similarities subtest of the WAIS-R.

Sometimes language is affected by a head injury. During interview attention is paid to the rate of speech, intonation, word usage, clarity of articulation, grammatical expression, length of sentences, and whether erroneous word use, such as gross mispronunciations or nonsense words, occurs. The Thurstone Word Fluency Test gives information about a patient's ability to generate words, while the Boston Naming Test measures one's ability to generate names for pictured items. The Reitan-Aphasia screening test provides a brief measure of various aphasia symptoms related to expressive and receptive language. Caution must be used in interpreting these test results because of the interaction effects of pre-existing language difficulties, as in learning disability.

Constructional abilities can be understood by means of both qualitative and quantitative results. The WAIS-R Block Design subtest requires an individual to reproduce a flat surface design when presented with cubes having different color designs to their surfaces. The qualitative measures include the apparent understanding of the "gestalt" of the design, while the quantitative measure is how many of the designs are completed and speed of problem solving. The Tactual Performance Test is more complicated in that the patient, while blindfolded, must place blocks of different geometric shape and size into spaces on a form board. Both of these tasks are often quite sensitive to the effects of various types of cerebral disorder.

Good information about the lateralizing effects of an injury may be obtained from tests of motor functioning if there are not significant peripheral injuries. The Grooved Pegboard Test, a measure of fine motor coordination, requires the individual to place grooved pegs into holes having varied orientation. This requires the patient to tactually perceive (and perhaps visually as well) the orientation of the groove of the peg in hand, visually comprehend the orientation of the groove in the pegboard, and then insert the peg. Performance is measured as time to complete the task and number of pegs dropped. The Finger Tapping Test, one of the more sensitive tests of cerebral dysfunction, requires the patient to depress the key on a manual counter for five trials of ten seconds duration, or five trials having a five point spread. Strength of grip is measured by a hand dynamometer. Steadiness may be quantified by using a hole-type steadiness tester. Comparison of results to normative data may suggest normal functioning, or lateralized or bilateral impairment. While all of these tests may be sensitive to cerebral dysfunction, they may also be affected by peripheral injury and medications.

Sensory perceptual examination may also provide information about materialization and localization of dysfunction. Sensory examination may reveal imperception, that is, failure to perceive sensory stimulation, or suppression, the failure to perceive stimulation on one side of the body under conditions of bilateral simultaneous stimulation. These, as well as tests of tactile form recognition and finger tip number writing recognition, require the patient to correctly perceive stimulation to the finger tips, and provide information about parietal lobe functioning in the absence of peripheral injury.

Emotional Adjustment

Emotional difficulties and personality changes may occur as a result of head injury and virtually every person who undergoes a neuropsychological evaluation should complete objective personality inventories. Brief scales exist for measuring depression and anxiety. The Beck Depression Scale, a transparent self report scale, might be replaced with the Hamilton Depression Scale, which requires examiner judgment. Anxiety may be measured by the State-Trait Anxiety Scale. The Minnesota Multiphasic Personality Inventory (MMPI or MMPI-2) is the preferred measure of personality characteristics because it also provides measures of profile validity and data useful in assessing symptom magnification or malingering (Pope, Butcher & Seelen, 1993). The Millon Behavioral Health Inventory provides information regarding personality characteristics as they affect reaction to illness or pain, and the Millon Clinical Multiaxial Inventory-II provides information regarding the nature of personality disorder, if it exists. Generally one would expect to find consistency across these different measures of symptoms and personality.

Summary

A neuropsychological examination, measuring level of intellect, academic achievement, attention, speed of processing, memory, abstraction ability, language functions, visuospatial and constructional abilities, various motor abilities, and assessment of psychological disturbance, is a more sensitive estimate of an individual's functioning than is a neurological examination in evaluating higher level cognitive abilities. Despite this sensitivity, there are many variables which may affect the data obtained and interpretation of those data. Just as an EEG may contain "noise", neuropsychological test data may contain the "noise" generated by examiner and patient variables. Examiner variables include various characteristics of the examiner and his skill in engaging the patient, administering and scoring tests, and the interpretation of results. Patient variables include the agenda or motivation of the patient (health versus litigation agenda), anxiety, depression, age, educational background, pain, medication or alcohol use, amount of sleep prior to the examination, and presence of various medical conditions. The sensitivity of the test results become much greater when the examiner considers the impact of these variables.

The neuropsychological examination then becomes an assessment having considerable validity and reliability for purposes of patient rehabilitation and litigation. For rehabilitation purposes it establishes a baseline for helping the patient become aware of (particularly in cases of denial) and more fully understand their residual deficits, use compensations to cope with these limitations, and develop skills to control anger or other changes which have occurred as a result of trauma. Re-examination may reflect the spontaneous restitution of function, document worsening of functioning as may occur in severely injured persons, or show non-improvement. For some the results of the neuro-psychological examination quantify the loss of function and may have considerable value for social security disability determination, worker's compensation benefits, and civil litigation. The test results also have the capacity to highlight an individual's residual capabilities, which can be useful when developingrehabilitation and treatment plans.

REFERENCES

Brittain, J.L., LaMarche, J.A., Reeder, K.P., Roth, D.L. & Boll, T.J. (1991). Effects of age and IQ on Paced Auditory Serial Addition Task (PASAT) performance. *The Clinical Neuropsychologist,* 5, 163-174.

Crosson, B., Novack, T.A., Trenerry, M.R. & Craig, P.L. (1988). California Verbal Learning Test (CVLT) performance in severely head-injured and neurologically normal adult males. *Journal of Clinical and Experimental Neuropsychology,* 10, 754-768.

Dalton, J.E., Pederson, S.L. & Ryan, J.J. (1989). Effects of post-traumatic stress disorder on neuropsychological test performance. *International Journal of Clinical Neuropsychology*, 11, 121-124.

Dacey, R.G., Jr., Vollmer, D. & Dikmen, S.S. (1993). In P.R. Cooper (Ed.). *Head Injury*, 3rd ed., 159-182. Baltimore, MD: Williams & Wilkins.

Ellis, D.W. & Christensen, A.L. (1989). *Neuropsychological Treatment After Brain Injury.* Boston, MA: Kluwer Academic Publishers.

Evans, R.W. (1992). The post-concussion syndrome. In R.W. Evans, D.S. Baskin, & F.M. Yatsu (Eds.). *Prognosis of Neurological Disorders*, 97-107. New York, NY: Oxford University Press.

Franzen, M.D. (1989). *Reliability and Validity in Neuropsychological Assessment.* New York, NY: Plenum Press.

Gennarelli, T.A. (1993). Cerebral concussion and diffuse brain injuries. In P.R. Cooper (Ed.). *Head Injury*, 3rd ed., 137-158. Baltimore, MD: William & Wilkins.

Goldstein, G. & Ruthven, L. (1983). *Rehabilitation of the Brain-Damaged Adult.* New York, NY: Plenum Press.

Goldstein, K. & Scheerer, M. (1941). Abstract and concrete behavior. *Psychological Monographs,* 53, (Whole No. 239).

Goldstein, S.G., Deysach, R.E. & Kleinknecht, R.A. (1973). Effect of experience and amount of information on identification of cerebral impairment. *Journal of Consulting and Clinical Psychology,* 41, 30-34.

Hartman, D.E. (1988). *Neuropsychological Toxicology.* New York, NY: Pergamon Press.

Heaton, R.K., Grant, I. & Matthews, C.G. (1991). *Comprehensive Norms for an Expanded Halstead-Reitan Battery.* Odessa, FL: Psychological Assessment Resources, Inc.

Helzer, J.E., Robins, L.N. & McEvoy, L.(1987). Post-traumatic stress disorder in the general population. *New England Journal of Medicine,* 317, 1630-1634.

Ivnik, R.J., Malec, J.F., Smith, G.E., Tangalos, E.G., Peterson, R.C., Kokmen, E. & Kurland, L.T. (1992). Mayo's older Americans normative studies: WAIS-R norms for ages 56-97. *The Clinical Neuropsychologist,* 6, Suppl., 1-30.

Ivnik, R.J., Malec, J.F., Tangalos, E.G., Petersen, R.C., Kokmen, E. & Kurland, L.T. (1992). Mayo's older Americans normative studies: WMS-R norms for ages 56-94. *The Clinical Neuropsychologist,* 6, Suppl., 49-82.

Johnson, D.A., Roethig-Johnson, K. & Middleton, J. (1988). Development and evaluation of an attentional test for head injured children-1. Information processing capacity in a normal sample. *Journal of Child Psychology and Psychiatry,* 29, 199-208.

Levin, H.S., Benton, A.L. & Grossman, R.G. (1982). *Neurobehavioral Consequences of Closed Head Injury.* New York, NY: Oxford University Press.

Lezak, M. (1983). *Neuropsychological Assessment* (2nd. ed.). New York, NY: Oxford University Press.

Litz, B.T. & Keane, T.M. (1989). Information processing in anxiety disorders: application to the understanding of post-traumatic stress disorder. *Clinical Psychology Review,* 9, 243-257.

Lynn, E.J. & Belza, M. (1984). Factitious post traumatic stress disorder: The veteran who never got to Vietnam. *Hospital and Community Psychiatry,* 35, 697-701.

Malec, J.F., Ivnik, R.J., Smith, G.E., Tangalos, E.G., Petersen, R.C., Kokmen, E. & Kurland, L.T. (1992). Mayo's older Americans normative studies: Utility of corrections for age and education for the WAIS-R. *The Clinical Neuropsychologist,* 6, Suppl., 31-47.

Matarazzo, J.D. (1990). Psychological assessment versus psychological testing. *American Psychologist,* 45, 999-1017.

McCaffrey, R.J., Hickling, E.J. & Marrazo, M.J. (1989). Civilian-related post traumatic stress disorder: assessment related issues. *Journal of Clinical Psychology,* 45, 72-76.

Miller, D.B. & Eckerman, D.A. (1986). Learning and memory measures. In Z. Annau (Ed.). *Neurobehavioral Toxicology.* Baltimore, MD: Johns Hopkins University Press.

Mirsky, A.F. (1987). Behavioral and psychophysiological markers of disordered attention. *Environmental Health Perspectives,* 74, 191-199.

Mirsky, A.F., Anthony, B.J., Duncan, C.C., Ahearn, M.B. & Kellam, S.G. (1991). Analysis of the elements of attention: A neuropsychological approach. *Neuropsychology Review,* 2, 109-145.

Mittenberg, W., DiGiuilio, D.V., Perrin, S. & Bass, A.E. (1992). Symptoms following mild head injury: expectation as etiology. *Journal of Neurology, Neurosurgery, and Psychiatry,* 55, 200-204.

Moon, G.W., Blakey, W.A., Gorsuch, R.L. & Fantuzzo, J.W. (1991). Frequent WAIS-R administration errors: An ignored source of inaccurate measurement. *Professional Psychology: Research and Practice,* 22, 256-258.

Perconte, S.T. & Goreczny, A.J. (1990). Failure to detect fabricated post traumatic stress disorder with the use of the MMPI in a clinical population. *American Journal of Psychiatry,* 147, 1057-1060.

Platt, J.J. & Husband, S.D. (1985). Post-traumatic stress disorder in forensic practice. *American Journal of Forensic Psychology,* 4, 29-56.

Pope, H.S., Butcher, J.N. & Seelen, J. (1993). *The MMPI, MMPI-2, & MMPI-A in Court.* Washington, D.C.: American Psychological Association.

Prigatano, G.P., Fordyce, D.J., Zeiner, H.K., Roueche, J.R., Pepping, M. & Wood, B.C. (1986). *Neuropsychological Rehabilitation After Brain Injury.* Baltimore, MD: Johns Hopkins University Press.

Raifman, L.J. (1983). Problems of diagnosis and legal causation in courtroom use of post-traumatic stress disorder. *Behavioral Science and the Law,* 1, 115-130.

Reitan, R.M. & Davison, L.A. (1974). *Clinical Neuropsychology: Current Status and Applications.* New York, NY: Wiley.

Reitan, R.M. & Wolfson, D. (1992). *Neuropsychological Evaluation of Older Children.* South Tucson, AZ: Neuropsychology Press.

Shum, D.H.K., McFarland, K.A. & Bain, J.D. (1990). Construct validity of eight tests of attention: Comparison of normal and closed head injured samples. *The Clinical Neuropsychologist,* 4, 151-162.

Slate, J.R., Jones, C.H. & Murray, R.A. (1991). Teaching administration and scoring of the Wechsler Adult Intelligence Scale-Revised: An empirical evaluation of practice administrations. *Professional Psychology: Research & Practice,* 22, 375-379.

Sparr, L. & Pankratz, L.D. (1983). Factitious post traumatic stress disorder. *American Journal of Psychiatry,* 140, 1016-1019.

Spreen, O. & Strauss, E. (1991). *A Compendium of Neuropsychological Tests.* New York, NY: Oxford University Press.

Thompson, G.N. (1965). Post-traumatic psychoneurosis-a statistical survey. *American Journal of Psychiatry,* 121, 1043-1048.

Tsushima, W.T. & Wedding, D. (1979). A comparison of the Halstead-Reitan Neuropsychological Battery and computerized tomography in the identification of brain disorder. *Journal of Nervous and Mental Disease,* 167, 704-707.

Harold H. Smith, Jr., Ph.D., ABPP

Located in Largo, Florida, Dr. Harold Smith is one of a few select psychologists holding the Diplomate in the specialties of Clinical Psychology, Forensic Psychology, and Neuropsychology. In addition to his Ph.D. in Clinical Psychology from the University of Southern Mississippi, he received an M.B.A. from the University of South Florida. He is licensed to practice psychology in Florida and North Carolina, and maintains a consultative and therapy practice. He has served as a Diplomate Examiner, officer in professional organizations, and as member and Chairman of the Florida Board of Psychological Examiners. Most recently he directed a hospital-based pain treatment program. He has extensive experience in the field of neuropsychology and has particular interests in the effects of closed head injuries, chronic pain, and malingering. He continues to publish and give invited professional addresses.

11

MALINGERING

Debra C. Price, Ph.D., David E. Raskin, M.D.
David R. Price, Ph.D.

The word "malinger" is derived from the French word malingre, which means "poor, weakly or ailing." The term evolved to indicate a situation wherein an individual intentionally produces false or exaggerated symptoms which do not, in fact, exist. The notion of manipulation for ulterior motives is included in definitions of malingering. For example, Webster's dictionary defined malingering as, "to feign illness in order to avoid duty," while Stedman's Concise Medical Dictionary indicated that to malinger was "to sham; to feign an illness, usually in order to escape work, excite sympathy, or gain compensation."

Malingering should be differentiated from other similar behaviors. Resnick (1984) describes these as dissimulation (the concealment or minimization of existing symptoms); partial malingering (the conscious exaggeration of symptoms which do exist); false imputation (the ascribing of actual symptoms to a cause consciously recognized to have no relationship to the symptoms); and factitious disorders (the voluntary production of symptoms for the purpose of assuming the patient role).

Faking the presence of mental illness or serious psychological disturbance has been present for centuries. Malingering mental illness was initially a problem in military and criminal settings. For example, individuals charged with crimes would fake psychological disturbance in order to avoid trial, sentencing, or execution. Likewise, individuals would fake mental illness to avoid the military draft and/or combat.

The presence of malingering has since spread to other arenas, and the methods and motivations to malinger are only limited by the individual's creativity and success. Sometimes individuals will malinger mental illness to obtain medications (particularly anxiolytic medications such as Valium and Xanax) or to obtain living conditions which they perceive to be better than their current ones; i.e., psychiatric hospital rather than being homeless.

Of particular concern to rehabilitation professionals, as well as to the insurance and defense law community, is the relatively recent phenomenon of malingering mental illness or organic disturbance to receive some type of financial compensation. Historically, objective physical symptoms of injury (loss of limb, fracture, laceration) were the stated consequences of injury. The objective nature of these symptoms left little room for doubt. In the late 1800's, however, the popular belief that concussion of the spine could result in nervous system abnormalities led to a new avenue for injury claims (Clevenger, 1889). This theory of nervous system changes following trauma to the spine opened the door to subjectively reported symptoms of injury rather than objective ones such as fracture. By the early 1900's, litigants started claiming such injuries as they sought compensation (Hamilton, 1906). By virtue of the nature of the claimed injury, they were not required to have accompanying objective symptomatology.

While awareness of malingering has been around for centuries, it was not until 1980 that the medical community formally recognized malingering and its impact on evaluation and treatment. The Diagnostic and Statistical Manual of Mental Disorders, published by the American Psychiatric Association, contains the classification system for the diagnosis of mental disorders. In 1980, the third edition of this manual (DSM-III) included malingering in this classification system. It was defined as, "the voluntary production and presentation of false or grossly exaggerated physical or psychological symptoms. The symptoms are produced in pursuit of a goal that is easily recognizable with an understanding of the individual's circumstances rather than of his or her individual psychology" (American Psychiatric Association, 1980, p. 331). The

DSM-III did not recognize malingering as a mental illness, but included it under the heading "Conditions Not Attributable to a Mental Disorder That Are a Focus of Treatment."

The DSM-III also included an index of suspicion to aid in determining the presence of malingering. On page 331 of the DSM-III it is stated, "A high index of suspicion of malingering should be aroused if any combination of the following is noted:

1. medicolegal context of presentation, e.g., the person's being referred by his or her attorney to the physician for examination;
2. marked discrepancy between the person's claimed stress or disability and the objective findings;
3. lack of cooperation during the diagnostic evaluation and in complying with the prescribed treatment regimen;
4. the presence of Antisocial Personality Disorder."

The 1987 revision of the Diagnostic and Statistical Manual (DSM-III-R) left these four elements unchanged. They were no longer described as an index of suspicion for malingering, but were presented with the advice, "Malingering should be strongly suspected if any of the following is noted" (DSM-III-R, p. 360).

Alan J. Cunnien (1988) also suggested a model for clinicians to follow to rule out malingering. Dr. Cunnien felt that the occurrence of any of the following, when accompanying psychological or physical symptoms, should alert a rehabilitation, treating or examining professional to assess and/or rule out malingering:

1. Involvement in civil or criminal legal action.
2. Potential for combat duty.
3. Lack of cooperation with examination and recommendations.
4. Complaints grossly in excess of physical findings.
5. Apparent environmental incentive for simulation of illness.

6. Suspicion of voluntary control over symptoms (such as they worsen when observed, are bizarre, and don't respond to treatment).

As mentioned previously, DSM (1980) defined malingering as, "the voluntary production and presentation of false or grossly exaggerated physical or psychological symptoms. The *symptoms are produced in pursuit of a goal that is easily recognizable with an understanding of the individual's circumstances* rather than of his or her individual psychology." Similarly, Dr. Cunnien has noted that a diagnosis of malingering must include an "obvious causal relationship between illness production and environmental incentives." Dr. Cunnien includes the following in a list of environmental incentives: avoidance of work, military service or incarceration; financial gain; avoidance of prosecution or execution; and, finally, the acquisition of drugs. Any one of these factors would be sufficient to establish as an environmental incentive to malinger.

Dr. Cunnien expresses concern about the incidence of malingering for financial gain, including avoidance of work as in Workers' Compensation or Disability claims. Related to this is the fact that both Dr. Cunnien and the Diagnostic and Statistical Manual include the context of litigation in their factors which should alert a rehabilitation, treating or examining professional to the possibility of malingering. It is not unusual to find that individuals malingering for financial gain and to avoid work may also malinger to receive prescribed drugs.

Related to the phenomenon of malingering for prescribed drugs is the issue of substance abuse. The Diagnostic and Statistical Manual has consistently included in the four factors in its index of suspicion of malingering the presence of an Antisocial Personality Disorder. This actually may not be as predictive as the presence of substance abuse/dependence. Substance abuse or polysubstance abuse often co-exists with an Antisocial Personality Disorder, and is often diagnosed along with the personality disorder. It should be noted, however, that antisocial behavior can be a consequence of substance abuse in the absence of an Antisocial Personality

Disorder. On page 344 of the DSM-III-R, it states, "When antisocial behavior in an adult is associated with a Psychoactive Substance Use Disorder, the diagnosis of Antisocial Personality Disorder is not made unless the childhood signs of Antisocial Personality Disorder were also present and continued into adult life."

The 1993 revision of the Diagnostic and Statistical Manual, DSM-IV, contains no changes with regard to the elements which should be examined to assess and/or rule out malingering. The manual continues to include the warning that "Malingering should be strongly suspected if any combination of the following is noted" (this refers to the four elements). This implies that if only one of the four factors is present, such as attorney referral for evaluation or treatment, then the presence of malingering should be strongly suspected. Unfortunately, this warning is too frequently ignored.

It would seem that the use of the aforementioned indices of suspicion would always allow the examining, rehabilitation, or treating professional to recognize malingering. This is not always likely to happen. Resnick (1988) stated, "No other syndrome is so easy to define, but so difficult to diagnose." Similarly, Asher (1972) noted, "The pride of a doctor who has caught a malingerer is akin to that of a fisherman who has landed an enormous fish." There are successful malingerers, and, since successful malingerers are not detected, the actual rate of successful malingering is not known.

There are a number of factors which contribute to a failure to correctly identify malingering. Traditional practice has often assumed the sincerity of patients in describing their symptoms and/or impairment. Treatment providers operate under the assumption that patients have a "wellness agenda" and that they will be honest in their pursuit of this. Given this assumption, the treatment provider does not often explore the possibility of distortion in the patient's report. In litigation, however, this distortion is all too common.

A second assumption found particularly in psychotherapy or counseling practice is that the truthfulness of the patient's self-report is of only secondary importance, since the primary focus of treatment is on process and not content issues. This assumption certainly reduces the likelihood that the presence of malingering is explored. It may also be noted that this assumption poses other problems given the increasing importance mental health systems have placed on assessment as a precondition in establishing proper treatment for the patient. As such, the assessment of patients' honesty and accuracy is of great importance.

The role of a treatment provider is often inconsistent with the role of one who is interested in ferreting out the possibility of malingering. The detection of malingering often requires a certain amount of tenacity and questioning of the patient's report. The treating physician is generally seen as a nurturing and supportive care-provider; this stance is generally necessary for a successful doctor-patient relationship. A doctor who appears to be distrusting of what his or her patient reveals would likely have difficulty keeping patients due to patients' perceptions that the physician is not caring.

This situation is compounded when the treatment provider is a rehabilitation or mental health professional who has had a long-term relationship with a patient. For this relationship to be successful, it is often necessary for the treatment provider and the patient to like and have positive feelings for each other. The health care provider, in essence, becomes an advocate of the patient, and wants to help the patient. Due to this position, the treatment provider often neglects to consider the possibility of malingering.

Regardless of the nature of the relationship with the patient, the average treatment provider does not spend the time and effort necessary to fully investigate the possibility of malingering. The average clinician, whether examiner or treatment provider, often is naive about the veracity of the claimant's self report, failing to assess the possibility of malingering enough (Binder, 1990, Reitan, 1992). Given the high rate of self reported symptoms associated with neuropsychological impairment in litigants (Lees-Haley, 1992), independent verification of the symptoms should always be pursued. This would include review of historical records, as well as conferring with other treatment providers the patient may be seeing. Heaton, Smith, Lehman, & Vogt (1978) suggest the best way to rule out malingering is when data from a variety of sources confirm the same results.

Clinicians are often at a disadvantage regarding making an appropriate diagnosis of malingering due to claimant deceitfulness and omission. The research is clear that clinical interviews are inadequate to assess malingering (Rogers, 1984). Additionally research has demonstrated that naive subjects can correctly self report symptoms of mild brain injury (Lees-Haley & Dunn, In press). In Lees-Haley and Dunn's study, 63.3% of subjects were able to correctly identify five or more of ten symptoms associated with mild brain injury. Malingering is most often discovered through careful review of historical records and detective work rather than clinical evaluation. The average treatment provider only has access to information which the claimant voluntarily provides.

It is difficult to malinger test results on objective physical diagnostic tests such as an electroencephalogram, magnetic resonance imaging technique, or bone scan. However, psychological and neuropsychological test results can be manipulated by subjects and "there is little to no scientific evidence that supports clinicians' ability to detect malingering with traditional measures of neuropsychological functioning" (Guilmette & Giuliano, 1991). Malingering may be successfully exhibited upon specific occasions (i.e., a short interview), but is extremely difficult to maintain across examiners, treatment sessions and modalities, or over time. Hence, it is often only demonstrable after careful record review with all of the claimant's examinations and medical or psychological data. Malingering may not be uncovered until the process of legal discovery begins and all relevant records are obtained for review.

Forensic Psychiatric Issues in Malingering

Malingering, as stated earlier in this chapter, represents a conscious feigning of symptoms in order to obtain understandable external gains. These gains include monetary compensation; certain kinds if responses from significant others; avoidance of unwanted events, such as being drafted; or escape from unwanted situations, such as being transferred from a jail infirmary to a mental hospital when an inmate pretends to be mentally ill.

The DSM-III-R distinguishes malingering from two other psychiatric concepts: 1) Conversion Disorder, and 2) Factitious Disorder. While malingering is not a mental disorder, conversion disorder and factitious disorder are psychiatric disorders.

According to the DSM-III-R, the essential feature of a Conversion Disorder is an alteration or loss of physical functioning that suggests a physical disorder(s), but that instead is apparently an expression of a psychological need or conflict. Symptoms of the disturbance are not intentionally produced, as in a Factitious Disorder or Malingering. Further, after appropriate investigation, the symptoms cannot be explained by any physical disorder or known pathophysiologic mechanism.

Factitious disorders are characterized by the repeated, knowing simulation of a physical or mental illness for no apparent purpose other than obtaining immediate medical or psychiatric treatment. To support their history, these patients may feign symptoms suggestive of a disorder, or may initiate the production of symptoms through self mutilation or interference with diagnostic procedures. The unique aspect of a factitious disorder is that the sole objective is to assume the role of a patient. Many of these patients make hospitalization itself a primary objective and often a way of life.

One distinction among the three concepts, malingering, factitious disorder, and conversion disorder, relates to whether or not an individual consciously produces symptoms. Another distinction is whether the symptoms are in order to gain understandable external things or whether the symptoms are produced in order to satisfy psychological needs which are unique to the individual.

The consciousness issue is a simple one in theory, but an imposible one to distinguish in practice. We have no real way of determining whether a specific problem such as paralysis of the hand is being willfully produced or not. We do have ways of determining whether the symptom is persistent, that is, through surveillance films or observation of the person in different contexts. It is possible to determine whether the symptom comes and goes. The assumption is that in the absence of persistent symptoms the particular problem, such as paralysis, is consciously produced. It is important to note that this may not always be the case. It is possible to have inpersistent symptoms which are still not willed. For this reason the distinction of conscious or willful symptoms versus unconscious or unwilled symptoms, although markedly helpful from a theoretical viewpoint, is one that is most difficult to identify in practice.

The issues of external understandable gains, often called secondary gains, versus internal primary gains is somewhat easier to determine. If, for example, a patient in a hospital consciously raises his thermometer's temperature in order to feign fever and we cannot figure out any monetary compensation or interpersonal response which might account for this, we are probably dealing with a factitious disorder which is related to the individual's psychological needs. For example, it may be that the individual came from a background where parents were physicians or nurses and the hospital environment has a peculiar meaning and security to that individual. Thus, the need to maintain a sick role in hospital bed is related to that need.

In summary, then, determining understandable secondary gain and distinguishing it from internal primary gain is a practical clinical task, whereas the issue of conscious versus unconscious production of symptoms is very difficult. The concept of conversion disorder is based upon an unconscious production of symptoms specifically related to an external stressor which produces a psychological conflict. This in turn leads to the unconscious expression of a symptom such as paralysis of the hand. Conversion disorder is a complicated diagnosis, is difficult to prove, and often has little jury appeal. Juries have difficulty understanding the complexity of the diagnosis and are skeptical about the unconscious production of symptoms. Conversion disorder, therefore, is a diagnosis which usually has little courtroom appeal and which disintegrates in the cross-examination of a competent attorney.

Factitious illness, in which a symptom is feigned consciously for internal needs, is a somewhat easier issue to present to juries. However, in most cases it is not a simple issue of primary or secondary gain, but rather a mixture of both. Once again, juries cast a skeptical eye on the concept of an internal need to produce symptoms versus all the other reasons people end up in litigation which involve monetary pay-off. The gist of the issue is that in the real environment of the courtroom, when considering the differential diagnosis of conversion disorder, factitious disorder, or malingering, the jury will naturally tend towards thinking of conscious symptoms for external reasons. That is, they will funnel most of the three disorders into a malingering mode. It is, therefore, extremely difficult to win the case if the diagnoses being put forward are either conversion disorder or factitious illness.

Turning now to the concept of malingering, there are several clinical forensic cues to malingering. These include, as has been stated in the first part of this chapter, a referral to a psychiatrist by an attorney rather than a health care provider, or a discrepancy between the patient's reports and objective findings. For example, in malingered gait disturbances, surveillance films often demonstrate normal gait while at the same time the patient stumbles around the psychiatrist's office. It is also common to find persons who are able to give detailed histories of their illness, their physicians, and their treatment but report problems when asked directly about their memory. They may also appear unable to answer questions which obviously tap memory functioning. Inconsistency, therefore, is a marker for malingered symptoms.

Another criterion is bizarre symptoms. In malingered memory disturbance the patient often complains of highly selective areas which are not consistent with organic memory disturbance. For example, patients will state that they can only remember certain years of their life or they can remember everything except for certain names or dates or they cannot recall bits of data such as the birthdate or the names of their children, yet at the same time they can repeat in great detail the history of their accident or injury. Since physicians, by their training and nature, tend to believe patients, doctors do not have a high index of suspicion for malingered behaviors. Often only trained forensic clinicians who are accustomed to assessing exaggeration and lying as part of the mental status look for these kinds of issues.

Another source for malingering will be found in the medical records. Medical records often reveal evidence completely inconsistent with the patient's description. Medical records may not reveal any evidence for unconsciousness or amnesia in a head injury while the claimant or patient reports definite periods of unconsciousness or retrograde or anterograde amnesia. The medical records will also reveal other sources of potential injury besides the event in question. Records from school or the military will also demonstrate baseline intellectual functions which are at the same level as post-injury testing or often below the level of post-injury testing. The claimants, however, often state that intellectual functions have deteriorated since head injury, even though the records do not bear this out.

Another source for the identification of malingering is the use of psychological testing. The Minnesota Multiphasic Personality Inventory (MMPI), and its revision, the Minnesota Multiphasic Personality Inventory-2 (MMPI-2), does help us in determining whether or not a person is taking the test in a totally credible way. There are now other tests which are being marketed which are more specific to the issues of malingered behavior and which promise to be helpful in the diagnosis of malingering.

In summary, the following points should be noted:

1. The distinctions between malingering, conversion disorder, and factitious illness, although useful in the clinical setting, fall to pieces in the amphitheater of the courtroom, and it is extremely hard to convince juries of the diagnoses of conversion disorder or factitious illness.

2. Malingered behavior is usually diagnosed by inconsistencies. These inconsistencies can be discerned in the clinical interview and are often found by detailed observation of the medical records or can be identified by psychological testing. The biggest block to identifying malingered behavior is the naive assumption by health care practitioners that patients are usually bent on telling the

truth, along with physicians' needs to side with their patients against what they often view as an onerous and diabolical insurance and courtroom system.

References

American Psychiatric Association. (1980). *Diagnostic and Statistical Manual of Mental Disorders* (3rd. ed.). Washington, DC: Author.

American Psychiatric Association. (1987). *Diagnostic and Statistical Manual of Mental Disorders* (3rd. ed., revised). Washington, DC: Author.

American Psychiatric Association. (1993). *Diagnostic and Statistical Manual of Mental Disorders* (4th. ed.). Washington, DC: Author.

Asher, R. (1972). *Richard Asher Talking Sense.* London, England: University Park Press.

Binder, L.M. (1990). Malingering following minor head trauma. *The Clinical Neuropsychologist,* 4, 25-36.

Clevenger, S.V. (1889). *Spinal Concussion.* London, England: F.A. Davis.

Cunnien, A.J. (1988). Psychiatric and medical syndromes associated with deception. In R. Rogers (Ed.). *Clinical Assessment of Malingering and Deception.* New York, NY: The Guilford Press.

Guilmette, T.J. & Giuliano, A.J.(1991). Taking the stand: issues and strategies in forensic neuropsychology. *The Clinical Neuropsychologist,* 5(3), 197-219.

Hamilton, J.E. (1906). *Railway and Other Accidents.* London, England: Bailliere, Tindall & Co.

Heaton, R.K., Smith, H.H., Lehman, R.A. & Vogt, A.T. (1978). Prospects for faking believable deficits on neuropsychological testing. *Journal of Consulting and Clinical Psychology,* 46, 892-900.

Lees-Haley, P.R. (1992). Neuropsychological complaint base rates of personal injury claimants. *Forensic Reports,* 5, 385-391.

Lees-Haley, P.R. & Dunn, J.T. (In press). The ability of naive subjects to report symptoms of mild brain injury, post traumatic stress disorder, and generalized anxiety disorder. *Journal of Clinical Psychology.*

Reitan, R. (1992). *Clinical neuropsychology: We've arrived, but do we want to stay.* American Psychological Association, August, 1992.

Resnick, P.J. (1984). The detection of malingered mental illness. *Behavioral Sciences and the Law,* 2(1), 21-38.

Resnick, P.J. (1988). Malingered psychosis. In R. Rogers (Ed.). *Clinical Assessment of Malingering and Deception.* New York, NY: The Guilford Press.

Debra C. Price, Ph.D.

Located in Greenville, South Carolina, Dr. Price is a Licensed Counseling Psychologist and a senior case analyst with the Insurance/Defense Network. She has had considerable clinical experience, having worked in private practice and with a pain treatment center. Her tenure at the pain clinic involved assessment and treatment of chronic pain patients, many of whom were workers' compensation cases. She has previously presented on the psychological management of the chronic pain patient, and has been published concerning diagnostic issues, most recently in the DRI special publication *Defending Cases Involving Psychological and Head Injuries* and on *Fictitious Closed Head Injuries* in *Claims.*

David E. Raskin, M.D.

See page 233

David R. Price, Ph.D.

See page 72

12

ECONOMIC ANALYSIS IN FORENSIC REHABILITATION

Jerome M. Staller, Ph.D.

Evaluating Loss

Making the Injured Party Whole

Tort law and rehabilitation facilities share a common goal: Both aim to return the injured party as closely as possible to pre-injury status. In tort law, this process is termed "making the plaintiff whole." The plaintiff is made whole, or as whole as possible, by an award of money if the defendant is found to be liable.

The amount of the monetary award is determined by either the judge or the jury — whoever acts as the "fact finder" in the case (some civil matters are heard by a judge without a jury). The fact finder decides what amount will be necessary to pay for rehabilitation costs where needed, to replace income lost (in the future as well as the past) as a result of the injury, and any other costs incurred as a result of the accident.

The economist's role in this process is to assist the fact finder in placing a monetary value on the injury. Each portion of injury to be compensated is referred to as "damages." The economist may be retained by the plaintiff, by the defendant or, in some instances, by the judge. An economist retained by the plaintiff normally provides a detailed report assessing the extent of damages. An economist retained by the defense normally critiques the plaintiff's economic report. Both are usually available to testify in the event the matter reaches trial. An economist may be retained by the court to help the judge better understand the damages issues before the court. Generally, the individual courts decide what the required qualifications of an expert will be. An expert witness is someone who has knowledge in a certain area beyond that of an ordinary person and whose knowledge will help the fact finder — the jury or, in cases without juries, the judge — better understand the facts of the case.

Economists who testify in court come from all types of backgrounds. Some are academics, some specialize in expert witness testimony (these are termed forensic economists) and some work in very specialized areas such as corporate finance and are retained in cases requiring this very specialized knowledge.

Elements of Damages

Damages encompass such costs as loss of past and future earnings, medical costs arising from the tort at issue, loss of household services and other, less tangible costs, such as the value of pain and suffering. The economist is concerned only with those elements of damages that can be reasonably valued. Punitive damages, meant to punish wrongdoers, are normally outside the domain of the forensic economist. Similarly, damages for pain and suffering are not amenable to economic analysis.

The basic elements of damages in personal-injury matters are fairly straightforward. They are:

- lost earnings
- lost fringe benefits
- lost household services
- medical costs

To assess damages in these areas, the economist considers a wide array of data and applies, in most instances, fairly sophisticated economic analyses. The required data falls into two main categories: statistical data relevant to the plaintiff's age, sex, race, job and family status and the economy; and data relevant to the plaintiff personally. Since both past and future loss is to be assessed, the economist must make some reasonable assumptions about the future: How much would the plaintiff have made had the injury not occurred? How will inflation affect future damages? What other factors will cause future damages to grow or diminish?

After the economist assesses probable future growth of income and the value of future damages, the damages figure must be "discounted," or reduced to present-day dollars. That is because dollars paid today to compensate for future damages can be invested and will earn money over time — a dollar paid today and invested can cover more than a dollar's worth of loss predicted to occur in ten years' time. The exact value of this "future" dollar depends on rates of interest and inflation, both of which must be considered by the economist.

The process of assessing damages can be as much an exercise in legal analysis as it is an economic effort. Throughout the process of calculating loss, likely growth rates and appropriate discount rates, the economist must adhere to the statutes and rules governing tort recovery in the relevant jurisdiction. Every jurisdiction has rules regarding how tort damages are to be assessed and what is recoverable. Rules vary from jurisdiction to jurisdiction, and a competent forensic economist must be aware of these sometimes obscure variations.

Medical Costs

In tort matters involving injuries requiring rehabilitation, medical costs will almost certainly account for a large proportion of damages. The services of several experts may be needed to accurately estimate the cost of ongoing medical care, necessary medical equipment, medicine and related costs.

First, a physician's opinion as to a future course of treatment and therapy is required — how much medication will be needed and what types of therapy and rehabilitation is needed. Beside drugs, medical procedures, therapy and rehabilitation, this category of damages includes the cost of special housing and transportation needs and the cost of nursing care, if needed.

Often, the physician who determines what the future care needs will be cannot estimate the cost of these needs. The opinion of a rehabilitation expert may be required. Typically, a rehabilitation expert puts together a "life care" plan detailing the treatment, equipment and services the plaintiff will require throughout his or her life expectancy. The rehabilitation expert then puts a dollar value on the services and equipment.

Here, it is important for the economist to know the frequency each item will be needed, how long the items will be required and, of course, the cost of each item. Once frequency, duration and cost is determined, the economist can project future medical costs by considering the effects of inflation and assigning a proper discount rate to the total, so that dollars payable for "future" damages today are reduced to present value.

Earning Capacity

Medical cost are not the only major element of damages in rehabilitation cases. Except in matters where the plaintiff is elderly or suffered from a preexisting condition limiting employment, the loss of earning capacity is a significant element of damages.

The measure of this element of damages is the difference between the plaintiff's earning capacity prior to the injury and the plaintiff's earning capacity after the injury. "Capacity" in this context is considered to mean demonstrated capacity. It is true that a plumber might become a brain surgeon, but for purposes of estimating damages the earnings of a plumber are the proper measure unless extremely compelling evidence exists showing that the transformation to brain surgeon is a distinct possibility.

Measuring Earning Capacity

The proper measure of lost earning capacity is a comparison of pre- and post-injury capacity. Three main variables must be considered:

- *Time* - How long would the injured person have worked had the incident not occurred? How long will the injured person work given the accident?
- *Money* - How much did the injured person earn prior to the accident, and how much would he or she have made had the accident not occurred? How much will he or she make given the accident?
- *Effort and ability* - Were there any indications that the injured person would have excelled at a given job or would have earned more due to any personal factors? Were there indications that the injured person would have made less than average, due to preexisting conditions, lack of skills or lack of motivation?

A great deal of data may be required to make a valid and accurate comparison of pre- and post-injury earning capacity. This data falls into two main categories — statistical data relating to the population at large and data specific to the plaintiff.

In general, the more specific the data is, the more accurate the economist's assessment of loss will be. It's helpful for the economist to know that the injured person is a 23-year-old male who had been working as a bartender prior to the injury. Various studies may indicate how much bartenders in the injured party's age, sex and race cohort will make. However, the economist will be able to provide a more accurate and complete earning-capacity assessment if the injured person's tax returns are also available. Such specific information will indicate exactly how much the injured party was making and might indicate how hard he was working.

Work-life tables are a statistical resource often used by forensic economists in determining future lost income. These tables, based on age, race and sex, indicate the plaintiff's work-life, or how long he or she might have been employed absent the injury. Active-life expectancy tables also offer insight into how long the plaintiff might have been employed, or would have rendered household services.

These tables, however, are poor measurements if there is any evidence that the plaintiff's work-life expectancy or active-life expectancy will diverge significantly from that of his or her age, sex, race and age cohort. Suppose a plaintiff suffered from a heart condition prior to a car accident. His work-life expectancy may have been drastically shorter than the average even before the accident, yet unless this is noted in an assessment of earning capacity, the earning capacity damages will be overstated.

Indeed, one of the most critical factors in determining post-injury earning capacity is the existence of any limiting condition — either physical or mental — that would tend to hinder earning capacity whether or not the injury occurred. This crucial point is sometimes overlooked, yet the plaintiff's condition prior to the injury can be the most significant element in earning-capacity assessment.

Vocational Assessment

Often, the economic assessment of earning capacity will be aided by an assessment from a vocational expert, who is able to offer an opinion on the types of jobs the plaintiff could have done had the injury not occurred, and the types of jobs open to then plaintiff given the injury. Frequently an injury will not affect the victim's ability to earn a living, but may require training in a new type of job. The vocational expert provides an outline of possible vocational alternatives in such instances.

One good indication of the plaintiff's post-injury earning capacity is the work he or she is actually doing. In many instances injured persons will find work at reduced earnings. Also, several studies exist that measure earning capacity in light of injury and disability.

The plaintiff's family situation may, potentially, be an indication of future earning capacity of a child. The child will have no employment history and, in all likelihood, there will be no clear indication of what profession the child will pursue. Here, in addition to scholastic records, the family may offer clues as to what career the child will pursue. It may be reasonable to assume that a child of a professional couple will go on to become a professional, for example. Also, where siblings have moved out of the household into careers, it may be reasonable to assume that the child will follow in the footsteps of brothers and sisters.

In the context of rehabilitation cases, it should be noted that cases where the plaintiff is totally disabled and will not improve are far easier to assess in terms of damages. The only assessment necessary is pre-injury capacity. Where there is some residual capacity, however, medical and vocational opinion must be elicited as to the extent of residual earning capacity.

Growth of Earnings

Over the course of a person's life, earnings will grow due to several factors. In assessing future lost earnings, the forensic economist must take such growth into account and estimate as closely as possible how earnings will grow.

Two main factors affect growth of earnings: inflation and productivity. Salaries rise due to inflation. It is the forensic economist's job to predict the course of future inflation and incorporate that estimate into future lost earnings calculations.

Another force acting on earnings is productivity, both personal and societal. Personal productivity can grow due to experience — the more experience we have, the better able we are to do our jobs and the more productive we become. Societal productivity increases due to such factors as the invention of fax machines and improvements in roadways that allow all U.S. industry to become more efficient. Both types of productivity increase must be factored into the earnings assessment.

The growth of an individual's income, of course, is mostly determined by that individual — if it can be demonstrated that the individual has worked harder than average in the past, it is likely that individual will earn more than average in the future.

Fringe Benefits

Many employees enjoy benefits over and above their base salaries. These benefits may include pension contributions made by the employer, life and health insurance, and profit sharing plans. The forensic economist must place a value on these fringe benefits, which may require complex calculations, especially in matters involving the value of pension benefits.

Household Services

Another element of loss in injury cases is lost household services — the chores a family member will do around the house for the benefit of other family members. Courts recognize that housework is just as important as outside work and should be compensated. Claims for household services are not limited to cooking, cleaning, child care and sewing, however. Efforts such as home carpentry, auto repair and lawn care can be as reimbursable. In most cases, the proper measure of these services is their replacement cost.

A CASE STUDY

Background

Cynthia was eight years old when she suffered traumatic brain injury in a head-on collision. She had been riding in the front seat. Her head hit the dashboard and she experienced an open depressed skull fracture to the left temporal region. She underwent emergency surgery.

Prior to the accident, Cynthia had been a straight-A student. She had completed second grade at the time of the accident. Cynthia's father is a high-school graduate employed as a supervisor for the U.S. Post Office. Her mother is also a high-school graduate who, prior to the accident, had been employed as an emergency medical technician.

Neuropsychological Report

Approximately one year after the accident Cynthia was examined by a clinical neuropsychologist. The neuropsychological and psychoeducational evaluation assessed Cynthia's current levels of cognitive, intellectual and emotional functioning.

The report on the evaluation noted that Cynthia's mother reported decreased attention span since the accident, memory problems and emotional and behavioral changes. She had no history of previous injuries and enjoyed good health prior to the accident.

Cynthia was given the Woodcock-Johnson Psychoeducation Battery academic tests as part of the evaluation. These tests were given to determine if Cynthia's traumatic brain injury affected her performance in school. The results suggested that there was significant difference between what she could be expected to achieve based on her past record and what she can expect to achieve based on her current performance and aptitude. The test results "strongly support the existence of cognitive deficits consistent with traumatic brain injury," the report noted.

Cynthia was also examined by a vocational evaluator employed at a rehabilitation center. This evaluation indicated that Cynthia's work opportunities given the accident will most likely be limited to occupations such as secretary, receptionist and similar jobs. Absent the incident, Cynthia had the capacity to complete college and pursue many different career paths, according to the vocational evaluator.

Earning Capacity

To determine what degree of earning capacity was lost as a result of the accident, the forensic economist first estimated Cynthia's capacity absent the accident. Operating under the assumption that Cynthia would have completed college, the economist examined U.S. Census data tracking average earning by age group for various levels of educational attainment.

Next, two assumptions were posited regarding the length of time Cynthia will work. First, an estimate based on continuous employment through to age 65 was calculated. Next, an estimate based on statistical worklife was calculated. The statistical worklife estimate was measured using data from the U.S. Department of Labor tracking rates of absence from the workforce by race and level of education — most workers experience some absence from the workforce at some point.

Two more assumptions were posited regarding Cynthia's earning capacity given the accident. Relying on the reports from the neuropsychologist and the vocational evaluator, the economist first calculated earning capacity under the assumption that Cynthia would graduate from high school and secure employment generating earning equal to those of an average high-school graduate. The estimate of these earnings is based on Census data.

Next, earnings were calculated based on survey data from the U.S. Department of Health and Human Services examining the effect of various disabilities on earning capacity. The assumption under this calculation was that Cynthia would complete high school but may suffer impaired earnings as a result of the brain trauma.

Medical and Ongoing Care

A report prepared by a rehabilitation expert estimated the costs Cynthia will incur over her lifetime for various evaluations, therapeutic modalities, medical procedures, medications, education needs and equipment. The costs were separated into three categories: ongoing medical care, ongoing education needs and one-time costs. Tables 12.1, 12.2 and 12.3 itemize the estimated costs.

TABLE 12.1 *Ongoing Medical Care*

Item	Duration	Annual Cost
Neuropsychological & Psychoeducational Testing	1992-2003	$742
Functional Capacity Evaluation	1992-2003	102
Cognitive Therapy	1992	2,000
	1993-2003	1,000

Continued

TABLE 12.1 *Ongoing Medical Care, continued*

Item	Duration	Annual Cost
Neurologist	1992-LE	$188
Psychotherapy	1992	3,000
	1993-2003	1,200
Serum Drug Level	1992-LE	45
Serum Liver Profile	1992-LE	80

TABLE 12.2 *Ongoing Education and Equipment Needs*

Item	Duration	Annual Cost
Private School	1992-2000	$8,850
After Hours Tutor	1992-2000	6,300
Specialized Post Secondary Training	2000-2004	1,600
Desktop Computer	1992-LE	458
Programs	1992-LE	125

TABLE 12.3 *One Time Costs*

Item	Total Cost
Vocational Evaluations	$1,871
Driving Evaluation	500
Behavior Modification	4,682
Vocational Counseling	5,367
Job Coach	62,166
Vocational Rehabilitation & Case Management	16,000
Recreational Therapy	2,000
EEG/Sleep Deprivation Study	375
Computerized EEG	1,300
Total One Time Costs	$94,261

TOTAL ECONOMIC LOSS

By subtracting all elements of earning capacity given the accident from earning capacity absent the accident, adding up all elements of medical and related costs (both one-time and ongoing) and reducing all future elements to a present value, the loss estimated under each alternative assumption was calculated. The results, as seen in Table 12.4, showed total economic loss (reduced to present value) ranging from $714,594 to $924,654.

TABLE 12.4 *Summary Table*

Assuming Full High School Earnings Given the Accident

Employment Status	Continuous Employment	Statistical Worklife
Earnings Absent the Accident	$1,255,518	$1,097,700
Pension Benefits	49,593	43,359
Value of Medical Costs	67,214	67,214
Value of Education & Equipment Needs	152,863	152,863
One Time Costs	94,261	94,261
Less:		
Earnings Given the Accident	815,113	712,653
Pension Benefits	32,197	28,150
Total Economic Loss	$ 772,139	$ 714,594

Continued

TABLE 12.4 *Summary Table, continued*

Assuming 18% Occupational Disability Reduction Given the Accident

Employment Status	Continuous Employment	Statistical Worklife
Earnings Absent the Accident	$1,255,518	$1,097,700
Pension Benefits	49,593	43,359
Value of Medical Costs	67,214	67,214
Value of Education & Equipment Needs	152,863	152,863
One Time Costs	94,261	94,261
Less:		
Earnings Given the Accident	668,393	584,375
Pension Benefits	26,402	23,083
Total Economic Loss	$ 924,654	$ 847,939

Jerome M. Staller, Ph.D.

Located in Philadelphia, Pennsylvania, Jerome Staller, Ph.D., is the founder of the Center for Forensic Economic Studies. The Center, founded in 1980, is a Philadelphia-based national firm staffed by full-time doctoral level experts providing economic and statistical analysis and testimony in all types of civil matters, including personal injury and wrongful death, employment and commercial damages.

Dr. Staller earned his Ph.D. in Labor Economics and Statistics at Temple University. He has served on several college faculties, including the University of Maryland and Pennsylvania State University. He is currently a faculty Lecturer in Law at Temple University School of Law. Prior to founding the Center, Dr. Staller was an economist at various federal agencies, including the Cost of Living Council and the Department of Labor. He was appointed by the court to analyze claims in the national Bendectin litigation.

INDEX